META MORPHOSIS WOMEN 40+

JAGUAR BEAST

WILL CASTILLO PETIT

Optimus4D Group Editions

First Edition: 11/12/23

Publisher: Optimus4D Group Editions

Cover Design: Elena Ciruelos

ISBN: [ISBN Number]

Printed in Spain

For permit requests, contact:

Optimus4D Group Editionsgrupoptimus@gmail.com

The information contained in this guide is for informational purposes only and should not be considered professional medical advice. Consult a health professional before beginning any training program or making significant changes to your diet.

www.optimus4d.com
Optimus4D Group Editionsgrupoptimus@gmail.com

Thank you for your support and enjoy your journey with the Jaguar Beast Metabolic Training Guide!

DEDICATION

To my valuable students, in the gym and life and partly also teachers in the joint search for well-being. Through more than 20 years, each of you, with your doubts, concerns and individual goals, has been my constant source of inspiration and learning. Thank you for trusting me as your guide on this journey towards the most important thing in life, because if we lose physical well-being everything loses value. This book is a testimony of our collaboration, where your needs have been the spark for the creation of knowledge. May these pages continue to be a source of motivation and direction on your paths to health and vitality. With deep gratitude and commitment, always here for you.

Will Castillo Petit

CONTENT

FOREWORD

I was very happy when they proposed the prologue for this book, I feel very comfortable representing it, I am pleased to present to you "Metabolic Training" of the JaguarBeast Method, an inspiring project that brings us closer to understanding more about the importance of care and the years go by and our actions must adapt. Author of the triple BestSeller "Jaguar Mentality and Strength". Will, did not come into my life at a very delicate moment, I was in total emotional imbalance, I was going to psychological help and the same doctor, upon seeing my progress, told me that her prescription was that I continue the training, today in this book you will be able understand how important it can be to "have" ourselves as a priority, take care of your health and of course be in the company of professionals such as the author of this book, who influenced the change of my life, my focus, and my physique

This is not the typical prologue, I am not a super professional and I endorse what this book says intellectually, it is about people, the beliefs and fears that hold us back, training, taking care of ourselves, respecting ourselves, it is not just about physical appearance and being beautiful. Which of course we love!!! And it's okay and you will achieve it, if you set your mind to it, this is about feeling good, about living and valuing each day as an opportunity .

For about 15 years now , I have witnessed and benefited from the positive impact of adopting not only physical activity habits but also being in the right place, making the most of my time effectively with training such as those presented by Optimus4D and its method. JaguarBeas, I'm honest with you, I would train more, but the trainer and author of this book does not advise me, but I will not get ahead of his lines.

The Optimus4D Tribe can become your ally, your group, your support, if you allow it, with its unique approach not only focusing on training efficiency, but represents an invitation to redefine the connection with exercise and vitality.

May this book propel you to a new stage on your journey towards the best version of yourself . Get ready for an interesting discovery, from the hand of this great professional and leader in his sector .

With the best of my intentions

Candela Lopez Sempere

Return to this sheet and write down the pages, points or term that you want to remember.

> **"If you want to achieve great things, you must be brave in the small things."**
>
> **-Dave Ramsey**

Chapter 1

ACTIVE LIFESTYLE CHALLENGES

Modern life presents us with countless challenges, and for many of us, time has become one of the most precious resources. People over 30 are often at the peak of their professional careers, some of us have family responsibilities and are involved in various daily activities. In this context, maintaining an active and healthy lifestyle can seem like a daunting task.

This method goes beyond these conflicts and although I have taken them into account, the most important thing is that it offers a solution for the hormonal changes that we face after the age of 30 with the decrease of important factors such as GH. fountain of youth, IGF-1, insulin and other factors that we will address and that we can positively enhance thanks to this metabolic activation training system in which my promise is that you will be able to obtain more and greater results for your life in less time, therefore faster and more effective and with less effort, but don't let this last phrase confuse you, it is not the typical TV sales advertising of getting strong while you are on the couch, of course it will require your commitment and effort but being in a quarter of the time than usual and needing fewer days, it is easier to maintain discipline and focus in an increasingly hectic world.

1.1 Lack of Time: Transforming Limitations into Opportunities

Facing the constant feeling of lack of time is a universal challenge. Work pressures, family commitments and daily responsibilities form a tangle that often seems to stifle the possibility of incorporating exercise into our lives.

However, various studies, such as the one carried out by the Institute of Applied Sports Psychology (Smith et al., 2018), suggest that changing the perception of time can transform limitations into opportunities.

By embracing the idea that every moment counts, we are not only re-defining our relationship with time, but we are also creating space for personal improvement.

I invite you to reflect with these lines on how conscious time management not only challenges perceived limitations, but also becomes the key to unlocking a path to lasting health and well-being.

> **Every minute spent on self-care becomes an investment in your own growth and transformation!**
>
> -Will Castillo Petit

1.2 Stress and Exhaustion:

A Journey Towards Balance

Discover how to transform stress and exhaustion into opportunities to revitalize yourself and move towards a state of sustainable well-being!

Busy, active lives often go hand in hand with high levels of stress and burnout. In this state, prioritizing personal well-being can be relegated to the background, even when understanding its importance.

I put it to you like this: the incessant whirlwind of

an active and busy life tends to color our days with high levels of stress and exhaustion. In these circumstances, prioritizing personal well-being is often a pending task, even when we recognize the liberating potential of physical activity in stress management.

Put yourself in Claudia's shoes. Nurse, mother of 4 children, 3 girls and a boy , a professional and committed mother, she loves her children and her job, she doesn't like to do things halfway and even though she has all the love in the world, that It does not free you from experiencing daily stresses. Her experience is a vivid example of the struggle with stress and fatigue that many of us face. At one point in her life (I could tell you the exact date) through the invitation of one of her daughters , Claudia discovered after trying a week training in Optimus4D, how the simple act of dedicating It's time for training not only mitigated stress, but also gave him a boost of daily energy and focus. And what seemed to take away a moment from his day to train, resulted in an engine that powered the rest of his day.

Without a doubt , exercise can be an effective antidote to everyday pressures.

Studies support Claudia 's experience . For example, research carried out by the Institute of Applied Psychology and Mental Health (Gómez et al., 2019) demonstrates how regular physical activity not only reduces levels of cortisol, the stress hormone, but also releases endorphins, significantly improving mood and ability to cope with stressful situations.

This information aims to help you understand how important it could be to maintain this type of routine in your life, not only for the physical and health benefits, but for everything that this entails in all aspects of your life, helping you to have more balance in the other areas, helping to overcome the negative consequences that arise from other circumstances, all these areas are important and define us and that is why we do not want to eliminate them, we want to improve them and to do so we must improve and control their effects at a metabolic and hormonal, perhaps you had not stopped to think about it, but without knowing this, you will have noticed that after exercising you notice an avalanche of relaxation and satisfaction, because you already know what has happened and it is just one of the points of this book.

Now I take you to explore the science that added to the personal experiences that underline the effectiveness of metabolic training as a beacon of balance in the midst of the choppy sea of modern life.

> **Although modern life may seem like a dark labyrinth, each step forward is a flash that dispels the darkness.**
>
> **-Will Castillo Petit**

1.3 Sedentary lifestyle

Technology and modern conveniences have led to a more sedentary lifestyle. Long hours in front of screens , combined with jobs that require little or no effort and lack of physical activity can contribute to long-term health problems, such as weight gain and decreased energy.

I really don't want to expand on this point, you just know it or you intuit it, if you are reading this book there are only 2 options for me, you are one of the warriors who makes life happen for you, you act and you are here to understand a little more everything that happens with your workouts , everything that you feel, or are you one of those who let life pass through you, which is neither good nor bad it just depends on what you want and if you are comfortable with that situation is perfect, but I understand that reading this is not where you want to be... I'll just tell you an open secret, when you are sedentary, that's when you least have time for yourself, you don't see the moment, you don't know how to do it and Guess what? That's how it will continue to be unless you get up, have a goal, take the first step and go for it.

You will soon discover that it was a big lie felt like a big truth and you know that I understand that it is also hormonal, bitches can make you feel like a super heroic or a super Incapable, without changing anything, just your hormonal state. And you are in control, you just have to activate the necessary mechanisms to start directing your life.

I'm talking to you about hormonal physical reactions, but in addition to being a physical trainer I am a wellness and mentality coach, I want to lift you to where perhaps you have never been or lift you back to where you were or how you felt in your youth, when you played sports, had fun and played in the streets or belonged to a team. Put the purpose in your mind, the idea of acting, and do it.

Generally everything begins with a thought, an idea, a desire, which makes us take certain actions that cause changes and in the case of sport, then it is these actions that give strength to our mind, making us stronger, positive and productive, so they complement and drive each other, many times the mind drives the body and other times the fact of changing, your pasture, its physical sensations, your strength, leads you to change your mind.

"You are what you are and you are where you are because of what you have put in your mind.   "You can change who you are and where you are by changing what you put in your mind."   - Zig Ziglar

1.4 Lack of Motivation The Struggle:

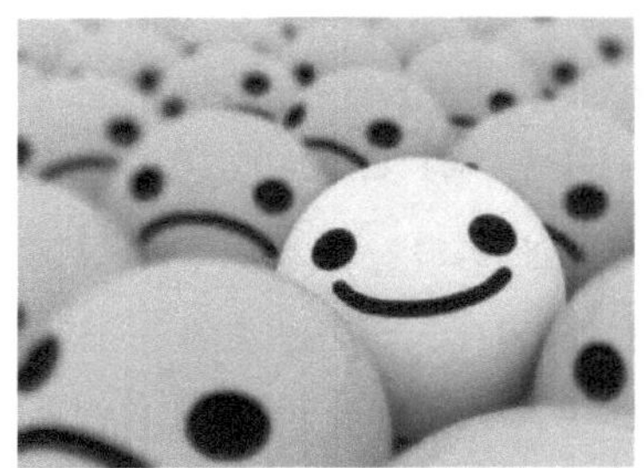

"Be miserable or motivate yourself, whatever you do is your choice" How do you want to be perceived?

Immersed in the complexity of our daily routines, we often face the constant struggle to find the necessary motivation to commit to ourselves, our health and well-being, we forget, as strange as it may seem logically, our own well-being, for some reason we know that to carry carry out our daily routine, work, partner, family, children, projects, etc. We can only be healthy, and it is what we pay the least attention to, we find ourselves most of the time deciding that we need motivation (reasons to take action), to move, train, avoid junk foods, and the truth is, regardless of the tools that we give you. offer in this chapter, I could end it with just this: What greater motivation do you need than to live your life to the fullest?

But let's face reality , we are not moved by common sense, which I usually say is anything but common, I don't remember where I read it but I never forgot it . The truth is that the demand for energy to overcome inertia and overcome fatigue becomes a persistent challenge.

However, consider Andrea , who shared her journey in search of motivation and discovered that metabolic training is not only a form of exercise, but an emotional catalyst that transformed her perspective on wellness. Through small achievements and celebrations, Andrea found the key to staying motivated : belonging to a tribe, the Optimus4D community.

The importance of belonging to a community

with similar objectives is revealed as a vital component to sustain motivation. The Optimus4D tribe not only provides support and camaraderie, but also establishes a space where individual achievements are celebrated as collective victories , of course dear reader this is a wide world and if you have the support of a community congratulations but if it is not my responsibility to offer you ours, it would not be coherent to tell you about a solution without telling you where to find it, so throughout the book you will see that you will be invited to be part of our community, and you will always be able to take the JaguarBeast method with you .

A study from the University of Applied Sports Psychology (Torres et al., 2020) supports this notion, highlighting how belonging to an active community significantly increases adherence to exercise programs.

Starting an exercise program can be challenging when motivation is low. The lack of quick results or the perception that exercise takes too much time often deters people from committing to a more active lifestyle.

That's why I invite you through practical strategies to find and maintain motivation on your metabolic training journey. From setting achievable goals to visualizing your achievements, you'll discover how each step brings you closer not only to your fitness goals, but also to a community that shares your vision and drives you toward success.

You are not alone in this journey! Join the Optimus4D tribe and discover the transformative power of pursuing common goals in the pursuit of an active and balanced life.

1.5 Realistic Objectives

The misconception that exercise requires long hours in the gym or participation in intensive programs can discourage those with busy schedules. Lack of information about more efficient approaches can lead to setting unrealistic goals.

I have seen how people who obtain results with this system, especially those over 40, become motivated, see great changes and then see themselves with more energy and strength and so perhaps it is a logical thought due to limited knowledge of how the body works. , these people begin to do more, train more, run, swim, marathons, Spinning , etc., suddenly they go from training 3 times a week for 18 to 45 minutes to being training every day for hours, and notice that their bodies begin to lose energy, they begin to gain weight and have physical discomfort.

They do not understand the mechanisms and increase the effort more and continue to lose form. I could give you dozens of these. For example, it is a mathematical result: the body is a machine.

Perhaps you have ever met a very athletic person and found them over the years who continue doing their sport but have lost their shape. This is recurrent in high-performance athletes and it is not a question of abandoning the activity, sometimes it is since that type of effort is not sustainable over time and I go further and tell you that it is not recommended either, and in the case of those who have not abandoned their activities and still lose their shape, I will tell you in this book what It is happening in broad strokes so that you can avoid them or get out of that situation.

On this occasion more is not better, so don't believe me when I tell you that you don't need ungodly hours of training, just see for yourself and if you can get something out of this chapter let it be: when you see yourself improving, changed, stronger , agile, energetic , don't fall into the mental trap of wanting to do more, just focus on improving what has already worked for you.

I have had thousands of students, they generally understand what I tell them, but we are human and we like to stumble, experiment for ourselves, and I can tell you thanks to these experiences that some of the people who have left to increase their effort, even At the moment I have not seen anyone who comes back stronger or better physically , much to my opinion on the contrary, especially in those over 35 years of age .

And this is not a situation that I like, nor do I use it to say: I told you so, since my desire is to instill sports habits in people whether or not they train in our club, the important thing is the example that they will transmit. in their environment, but sometimes cases like the one I will tell you happen.

I will give you the example of Silvia , one of our great partners , dynamic , involved and an example to follow . Silvia achieved an impressive change in her physique , even people asked me if she had had surgery , it was fantastic, she was full of energy. , vitality, something that you will also experience if you apply our training method.

Our friend fell apart and he wanted to take advantage of all his new vitality, he continued training with us but since we only trained for three days he joined another gym to do another 3 of something similar called crosstif or something like that, sometimes both routines on the same day, he did extensive bike routes all On the weekends and whenever she could she went jogging to accompany other friends . She couldn't explain how she started to gain weight. to have joint problems , fluid retention and even hormonal disorders (you will soon understand why) , this situation led her to try harder to return to her physical shape but it was getting worse, the body for some reason that she did not understand to So , to be honest, I tried to explain it to him on some occasion but due to mysteries of the human being at that time he did not understand me. I suppose that everything has its moment... I hope and trust that if you are reading this, it is because this is yours that you understand this reading and it will be useful to you .

So, dear friend, this example and everything I mentioned at the beginning of the chapter should give you peace of mind if you are not a sports lover "Even" you do not need a great sacrifice or time translated into an hour at the gym, therefore not only do you not You need to put in hours of training but it is also counterproductive unless you are 16 years old and your body can withstand everything that is thrown at it, but here I am writing about my experiences and you reading I think we have already passed that stage, now let's enjoy the advantages this.

For me in particular, this physical wisdom is a blessing that we require less effort for less time to obtain better results and of course grateful that there are studies that confirm it, although I am honest with you when you grow up surrounded by sports and athletes, you do not need studies to Realizing it, you end up connecting the dots, but I like to put words into these processes so that you can also understand it.

> **"Do not underestimate the power of taking advantage of other people's experience; every mistake avoided is a shortcut on the path to success."**
>
> **Will Castillo Petit**

1.6 The Need for Practical Solutions

Amidst these challenges, there arises a dire need for practical and efficient solutions that harmoniously integrate with a busy lifestyle. By creating the Optimus4D system and its in-person and online training system, it not only recognizes these challenges, but also offers an effective response to overcome them.

It is clear that you can find other training that uses these principles to achieve metabolic training, so you can train with whoever you want, wherever you want and whenever you decide, but I cannot speak to you for anyone else if I give you guarantees for others, I give you this information is valid . wherever you are and on the other side of the world, but it would be absurd not to offer you a solution or tool to do it, that's why I present to you JaguarBeast and The Optimus4D Tribe

<u>Scan the Code or click on it </u>to access the Optimus4D Online Tribe, I'm looking forward to meeting you, I'll see you inside

C onclusion of Chapter 1

As we embark on the exploration of the challenges inherent to an active lifestyle, we recognize that time limitation is not the only barrier to overcome, but rather a fundamental aspect for the design of practical solutions adapted to everyday demands. Over the next few sections of this book, we will dive into solving these challenges and venture together on the path to lasting, attainable well-being.

Get ready to experience a significant transformation in your approach to exercise and discover how this path can positively shape your life!

Chapter II

Hormonal Impact of Training
Metabolic JAGUAR BEAST
In Women 40 +

Metabolic training is revealed as a transcendental element, especially for women over 40 years of age, where the hormonal experience takes on different nuances and demands more specific attention.

The benefits of physical activity and exercise on women's health are indisputable, a fact that is supported by strong scientific evidence in more than twenty-five medical conditions, including cardiovascular disease and premature mortality.

Although hormonal similarities remain, the particularities of our journey require a more detailed approach. My personal experience, starting my own transformation of changes in the behavior of my body at the age of 30, motivated me to adjust my training methods to offer my clients not only the best, but the most appropriate.

What the Jaguar Beast method will do for you is trigger a series of hormonal responses that go beyond simply burning calories. This chapter will explore how this specific training approach can positively influence the key hormones that play a crucial role in the well-being and health of women at this stage of life.

> **"Goals are the map, dedication is the vehicle, and success is the destination."**
>
> -Will Castillo Petit-

2.1 Estrogen:

The Key to Female Vitality

The hormone estrogen, essential for female well-being, undergoes natural fluctuations as we age. However, various studies, such as the one carried out by Breast Cancer Res., 17 (2015), suggest that metabolic training can be a positive catalyst for estrogen levels. Intensive and focused routines not only impact calorie burning, but also awaken specific hormonal responses, contributing to the vitality and hormonal balance of women over 40 years of age.

The protective effect of practicing regular physical activity in preventing health problems such as cancer has been well studied. Research shows a 25% reduction in the average risk of breast cancer in physically active women

And what brings us together, detailed research reveals that metabolic training, characterized by intense and precise sessions, acts as a stimulus to increase estrogen levels. Each session triggers internal mechanisms that prompt the body to produce more of this key hormone.

Incorporating Elements of Strength and High Intensity Cardio:

Metabolic routines don't just focus on duration, but quality and intensity. T he strategic combination of strength exercises and high-intensity cardio creates an environment conducive to stimulating estrogen production. The challenging resistance and intense bursts in cardio generate specific hormonal responses that contribute to hormonal balance and vitality in women over 40.

Counteracting the Natural Decrease in Estrogen Effectively:

As we age, estrogen levels naturally decrease, but metabolic training offers an effective response. As we delve deeper, you'll understand how these routines not only keep hormone levels within a healthy range, but also counteract the natural tendency of decline associated with age.

Promoting Vitality, Hormonal Balance and Energy:

The connection between metabolic training and female vitality manifests itself in tangible results. When you immerse yourself in this type of routine, you explore how this form of exercise not only stimulates the production of estrogen, but also translates these elevated hormonal levels into concrete benefits: greater vitality, hormonal balance and a renewed dose of energy to face each day and of course I am going to talk to you about endorphins that go one step further in the benefits observable to the naked eye also in triggering biochemical processes that translate into a better attitude toward life .

Revealing Conclusions:

In summary, this chapter distills the essence of how metabolic training becomes a catalyst for maintaining and enhancing female vitality. From hormonal stimulation to tangible physical results, this training approach offers a solid path toward optimizing the overall health and well-being of women over 40.

And while you begin to recognize concepts, I invite you to immerse yourself in the very essence of how each training session contributes not only to burning calories, but also to revitalizing your internal vitality.

Welcome to the JaguarBeast experience, where every effort counts and every repetition boosts your energy and vitality!

> **"On the journey of life, you are not alone. Learn from the setbacks and achievements of those who come before you, and turn their experience into a map for your own journey."**
>
> **-Will Castillo Petit**

> **This chapter will fascinate you if you were looking for the icing on the cake to love metabolic training, I present to you the fountain of youth, I invite you to dive into its waters**

Chapter 2.2

Growth Hormone (GH)

Renewing Vitality in Women

Growth Hormone (GH), widely recognized as the "fountain of youth" for its crucial role in cell regeneration and tissue maintenance, takes center stage in this intriguing chapter. Research, such as those conducted by Kraemer, et al. (1990), provide insights into the connection between metabolic training and GH release, revealing how this approach to exercise may be a key driver in maintaining vitality and health in women over 40.

The Science Behind the GH Stimulus:

Revitalizing Feminine Energy

In this chapter, we explore how metabolic training becomes the driving force for releasing Growth Hormone (GH), using artistic analogies such as ballet and symphonies to illustrate its effectiveness.

By diving into Kraemer and his team's study, we unraveled the mechanisms that link these specific routines to GH release, revealing a deeper strategy than might initially appear.

Imagine training sessions as ballet pieces or symphonies, where meticulous planning, especially that which boosts the heart rate and challenges the muscular system, is revealed as an effective tactic to release GH. Through research-backed examples, we understand how each movement and tactical choice triggers specific hormonal responses.

Visualize a coordinated ballet, where each dancer performs her role with precision, achieving a synchronized hormonal response. This process, from the activation of cellular receptors to the stimulation of specific glands, gives us a clear vision of how our body, immersed in metabolic training, executes a winning strategy to enhance the internal "fountain of youth."

Get ready to immerse yourself in this training strategy, where science becomes an exciting game, signaling us that we are on the right path and using our time shrewdly. We are going to bring this story to life, where our body, like a ballet company or an orchestra, executes a masterful tactic to boost the release of Growth Hormone (GH). Each movement and tactical choice contributes to a unique strategy that awakens a complex and harmonious hormonal response. Your well-being will reach new heights as each training session becomes a strategic game that elevates your internal source of feminine vitality.

GH as a Pillar in Muscle and Bone Health:

The focus of this chapter extends beyond simply recognizing the connection between metabolic training and GH.

One of the most exciting discoveries during my research was understanding the vital role of GH in preserving muscle mass and bone health in women over 40. Now you will understand how each training session is not only an opportunity to burn calories, but also a stimulus for the release of GH, a process that promotes muscle toning, the reduction of body fat and the maintenance of strong bones.

Let's continue weaving the hormonal processes, observing how they are produced and intertwined, to offer you clarity on why it is so effective for you to adopt this training system: Metabolic Training, your Source of Internal

Vitality.

At this point, my goal is to provide you with a detailed vision based on scientific research, but in a simple way. I do not intend to offer you a clinical trial, but rather to give you the spark necessary to begin your search for all these benefits, without overwhelming you with an extensive dictionary of unnecessary terms. This chapter guides you through how metabolic training becomes a crucial ally in maintaining the internal "fountain of youth."

It's no longer just about recognizing terms, but about understanding how each exercise choice, each intensity, and each training session become active contributors to stimulating GH release.

This knowledge not only expands your understanding of the connection between metabolic training and GH, but also empowers you to make the most of every minute of exercise in the pursuit of long-lasting vitality.

Shocking Conclusions:

At this point, I hope you are clear on the idea of not only how the relationship between metabolic training and GH benefits, but how this approach to exercise becomes a catalyst for maintaining the internal "fountain of youth" in older women of 40.

Every conscious choice of movement becomes an investment in maintaining vitality and health as you move through life. Prepare to take with you not only the knowledge, but also the specific actions that will contribute to your overall well-being.

Welcome to the world of the possible, especially to the JaguarBeast Method and the Optimus4D Tribe, where inner youth is renewed with each repetition and where metabolic training stands as the indispensable ally for lasting health!

"Your vision and your actions are the architects of your destiny; make the first great and improve the second; build with wisdom."

-Will Castillo Petit

2.3: Cortisol

Navigating the Waters of Hormonal Stress

Cortisol, known as the "stress hormone," plays a crucial role in the body's response to stress and is associated with various physiological functions. Chronic stress, such as that experienced by many women around age 40 due to family responsibilities, work, projects and studies, can have adverse effects on health. However, exercise, particularly certain types of training, may have benefits in cortisol management and stress response. Here are some considerations backed by studies:

1. Effects of Exercise on Cortisol:

Physical exercise, especially aerobic and resistance exercise, can help modulate the cortisol response. Studies have shown that regular training can lead to an adaptation of the hypothalamic-pituitary-adrenal axis, which regulates the release of cortisol, resulting in a more attenuated response to stress.

2. Intensity and Duration of Exercise:

The intensity and duration of exercise can influence how it affects cortisol. It has been observed that moderate and moderate-intensity exercise can have positive effects on the regulation of cortisol, while extremely intense or prolonged exercise could temporarily increase the levels of this hormone .

This reaction, among others, could perfectly explain the reactions to which people are exposed, as in the case that I explained to you before about our student Silvia. It is a very powerful hormone that is generated in response to various situations in our lives, such as above. We can provoke it actively and in large quantities, and physical activity that is positively associated with stress regulation could turn it around "whether we understand this process or not . " I comment on it in the next point.

3. Exercise for Stress Management:

CORTISOL AND ENDORPHINS

Exercise has emerged as a highly effective strategy in stress management, playing a fundamental role in emotional balance and mental well-being. One of the main reasons behind this effectiveness lies in the release of endorphins, neurotransmitters known as the "happiness hormones." This phenomenon, intrinsically linked to physical activity, not only counteracts the negative effects of chronic stress, but also positively influences levels of cortisol, the stress hormone.

Endorphins, secreted by the central nervous system and the pituitary gland, act as natural pain relievers and generators of well-being. Its release is enhanced during and after exercise, creating a feeling of euphoria and relief. This direct impact on mood contributes significantly to the reduction of perceived stress.

When we engage in physical activities, whether through metabolic training like in the Optimus4D tribe , yoga, running, or any form of exercise, a cascade of neurochemical events are triggered. Intense physical activity stimulates the production and release of endorphins, which bind to opioid receptors in the brain, reducing the perception of pain and generating a feeling of well-being.

Additionally, the mood enhancement associated with endorphins may have a positive impact on cortisol regulation. Cortisol, when chronically elevated due to prolonged stress, can have adverse health effects such as suppression of the immune system, increased blood pressure, and accumulation of abdominal fat. The ability of exercise to counteract these effects by influencing the release of endorphins becomes an essential component in maintaining hormonal homeostasis.

In short, regular exercise not only provides

tangible physical benefits, but also acts as a powerful stress regulator. The release of endorphins, as a direct response to physical activity, not only improves mood, but also contributes to the effective management of cortisol, thus strengthening the connection between exercise and overall health.

4. Resilience Exercise:

Hear the drum, some studies suggest that regular exercise can contribute to stress resilience, meaning people can better handle the stressful demands of daily life. This is especially relevant if you face multiple responsibilities.

5. Individual Considerations:

In summary, regular exercise, particularly moderate intensity exercise, may be beneficial for women who experience chronic stress due to the multiple responsibilities associated with age and life circumstances.

However, individualization of the exercise program, considering health and personal preferences, is essential.

It is always advisable to consult with a health professional before making significant changes to your exercise program, especially in situations of chronic stress.

Concrete Examples

As you may have already appreciated, my goal is not only for you to explore the theory behind hormonal stress and metabolic training, but also for you to immerse yourself in the palpable reality of real individuals who have transformed their lives through high-intensity routines. Through inspiring stories, you will learn stories of triumph over chronic stress.

I'm talking to you about Verónica , a store clerk, with the added bonus of being in charge of warehouse management and generally long hours and constant work pressure. Through metabolic training, Veronica Not only did he manage to maintain his health and exceptionally regain his physical fitness , but he also experienced a notable decrease in cortisol levels, allowing him to face daily challenges with greater mental clarity.

María, mother of three children, found metabolic training a refuge to manage everyday stress. Her high-intensity sessions not only provided her with a healthy emotional outlet, but also contributed to maintaining her cortisol levels in an optimal range, and of course recovering her optimal physical condition after the last birth, improving her general well-being and her ability to manage family demands .

You could identify with some of those cases , but the goal is for you to know that at any given moment we can all feel the effect of this hormone overflow and affect us.

These are just two examples of how real people, facing different contexts and challenges, have embraced metabolic training as a vital tool to manage hormonal stress.

From gym workouts to JaguarBeast sessions at home, every success story supports the claim that metabolic training is not just a set of exercises; It is an active strategy to maintain hormonal balance and, therefore, a healthier and stress-resistant lifestyle.

Prepare to absorb these examples and live them out in your own experience and discover how metabolic training becomes a transformative tool for those looking to not only improve their fitness, but also successfully navigate the waters of hormonal stress.

Keep exploring the wonders that this path has in store for you!

Each Training Session

as Active Strategy:

Imagine for a moment: each training session is not just a routine; It is an active strategy to counteract the harmful effects of chronic stress. Every repetition, every weight lift, becomes a step towards hormonal balance and the preservation of your health. Through vivid narratives, you'll delve into the very essence of how metabolic training becomes an active defense against the ravages of persistent stress.

Get going and discover how metabolic training becomes your compass to navigate hormonal stress.

> **"Success is not the key to happiness. Happiness is the key to success. If you love what you do, you will be successful."**
>
> -Albert Schweitzer

Meet the Optimus4D Tribe! You will love her!!!

2.4: Insulin

Optimizing Metabolic Sensitivity

When we refer to insulin sensitivity, we are talking about the body's ability to respond efficiently to insulin, a hormone crucial for regulating blood glucose levels.

Insulin resistance, common with aging, means that cells do not respond properly to insulin signals, which can lead to a buildup of glucose in the blood and the development of metabolic problems.

Metabolic training, according to studies such as that of Francois, et al. (2019), emerges as a fundamental ally to improve this sensitivity. How does this happen?

1. Efficient Glucose Mobilization:

During metabolic training sessions, particularly those that integrate high-intensity and resistance exercises, muscles experience substantial activation.

This degree of muscle activation generates a higher energy demand, which, in turn, drives the efficient mobilization of glucose for immediate use. In this process, the body optimizes the use of resources, allowing more effective management of glucose, which is mobilized to satisfy the specific energy demands generated by high-intensity exercise and muscular resistance.

This phenomenon highlights the body's adaptability to respond effectively to changing demands during metabolic training, thus demonstrating how these sessions not only stimulate muscle activation, but also trigger precise metabolic processes to maintain a constant and adequate energy supply.

2. Stimulus for Muscle Cells:

The Regulatory Power of Insulin

Within the fascinating scenario that constitutes metabolic training, an intricate connection between physical activity and glucose regulation is revealed. This process is not limited to a momentary response; It is a sustainable transformation in the way our muscle cells interact with insulin.

When we perform metabolic training sessions, muscle cells are activated in an exceptional way. This cellular activism becomes a constant stimulus that awakens the sensitivity of these cells to insulin. This essential phenomenon Improves the body's ability to regulate circulating glucose levels.

The key lies in consistency. Every repetition, every exercise, and every moment of effort translates into a signal to your muscle cells: it's time to pay attention to insulin. This process is more than just a response; It is a continuous adaptation that is rooted in cellular memory.

Research, such as that of Francois et al. (2019), support the idea that metabolic training not only optimizes insulin sensitivity, but also improves the ability of muscle cells to efficiently uptake glucose.

Imagine these muscle cells as diligent learners, each training session providing them with a lesson in which they hone their ability to interact with insulin.

As you persist on this journey, your body becomes a masterful master of glycemic self - regulation.

With this fascinating information I hope you will weave together the molecular and cellular journey you experience when adopting metabolic training. Each repetition is not only a physical effort; It is an instruction encoded in the language of cells, a lesson that leads to renewed harmony between insulin and glucose.

the regulatory potential of insulin through consistency and commitment in your regular metabolic training practice !

Be optimus4d my friend

It flows like water surrounding the rocks in a river , they don't try to cross them... To you 1) What stops you? 2) Is it real? 3) does it matter more than living?

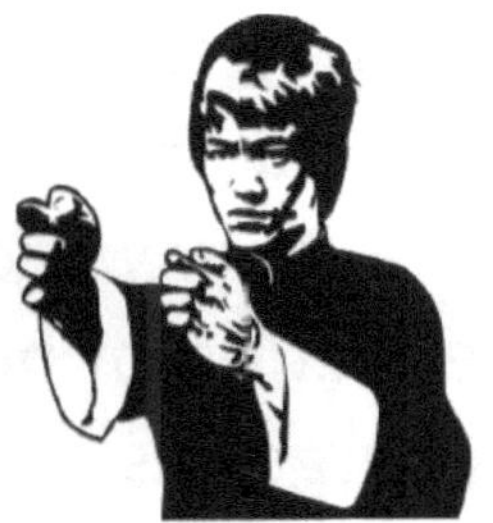

3. Reduction of Body Fat:

The Secrets Behind JaguarBeast for Reduced Body Fat

Decreased insulin resistance is associated with reduced body fat, an aspect that metabolic training effectively addresses by promoting fat loss and gains in lean muscle mass.

Get ready to immerse yourself in the amazing journey towards a body transformation that goes beyond your conventional expectations. I unravel in a few words the mysteries surrounding the reduction of body fat and how metabolic training emerges as an undisputed hero in this narrative.

Imagine this process as a choreographed ballet, where insulin resistance and body fat dance in harmony. Metabolic training, by decreasing insulin resistance, unleashes a domino effect on your body composition. We're not just talking about weight loss here; We are talking about a total transformation.

Each training session is not only a step towards strength and endurance; It's a neat twist in the plot of your relationship with body fat. And I have to mention again the study by Francois et al. (2019), because it also walks us through the intricate movements of how metabolic training not only promotes fat loss, but also embraces building lean muscle mass.

Now, visualize each repetition as a progression in the script of your own transformation story. Each exercise that is indicated to you is not only a physical challenge; It's an epic moment when insulin resistance gives way to fat loss. The stage is set for you to become the protagonist of your own body change narrative.

You experience or will experience how these workouts plus the social benefit of being short, targeted and maintaining their effects for hours, so only 3 days is an ideal scenario, we will take you with these workouts beyond conventional expectations and you will immerse yourself in a transformative experience that challenges the limits of the ordinary.

So, get ready to unleash a wow effect on your journey to body fat reduction that will resonate with every fiber of your being.

Welcome to the metabolic revolution where results go beyond what you thought you were capable of achieving!

4. Metabolism Optimization

Metabolic training not only impacts during the exercise session; Its influence extends to the post-workout period, where an optimized metabolism is maintained.

This continuous process helps to maintain stable glucose levels, thus promoting greater insulin sensitivity on a daily basis.

In conclusion, it is okay and important that you understand how it works, so that by understanding you can evaluate how each exercise choice in metabolic training generates tangible benefits for your metabolic health, being aware of this and as a person who values their life and well-being, this It should translate into one more incentive when getting ready to train and if you still don't love training and you're wondering, why do I do this? Is it worth the effort? Remember that there is something more important than your laziness or your doubts and that should win over the magnetic force of the sofa.... and that is the best version of you.

Get ready to explore how each session not only burns calories, but is also an active strategy to optimize insulin sensitivity and improve your overall well-being!

> **"Don't worry about failures, worry about the possibilities you lose when you don't even try."**
>
> **- Jack Canfield**

1. Reinforced Bone Health

The Hidden Gem for Vitality Throughout the Years

In this deeper exploration into the benefits of metabolic training, we unearth a hidden gem: its significant impact on bone health, a crucial consideration, especially as we cross the threshold of years.

One of the most notable benefits of metabolic training in relation to estrogen in men is its positive impact on bone health.

Specific exercises, such as those involving weight-bearing and resistance, stimulate estrogen production, which contributes to greater bone density and reduces the risk of osteoporosis.

Imagine each repetition as a foundation builder for your bone strength. Studies, such as the one carried out by Schneider et al. (2015), illuminate the intricate connection between specific metabolic training exercises and estrogen production. This hormone, which as we mentioned at the beginning and is well known decreases over the years , will emerge as a valuable defender of bone density , without forgetting the other benefits .

Every load and resistance applied during your training session is not only a challenge for your muscles, but also an active strategy to support your bone health.

Enjoy this fascinating journey discovering how metabolic training becomes an ally in the fight against the loss of bone density associated with aging.

It is crucial to understand that this benefit not only resonates in the present, but establishes a solid foundation for the future. In each circuit you perform, you are building your bones' resistance against the passage of time. This chapter reveals the vital role of metabolic training in reducing the risk of osteoporosis and promoting bone vitality that lasts over the years.

So get ready to celebrate this essential benefit of metabolic training, where every movement is an investment in your bone strength. As you progress on your journey, keep in mind that you're not just building muscle; You are strengthening the foundations of a full and active life as the years go by .

Welcome to the metabolic revolution that nourishes every aspect of your well-being!

2. Promotion of Cardiovascular Function

Hormonal balance, including adequate estrogen levels, plays a vital role in cardiovascular health.

Metabolic training routines, by influencing these hormonal levels, contribute to maintaining optimal cardiovascular function, reducing the risk of heart disease.

Specific Example 1: Resistance Weight Lifting :

Resistance training, such as weight lifting, activates muscles intensely, stimulating estrogen production.

This hormonal increase not only strengthens muscles, but also contributes to maintaining a proper hormonal balance for health.

Specific Example 2: High Intensity Training (HIIT) in Optimus4D (HIPT)

HIPT (high intensity power training) sessions, characterized by short but intense bursts of exercise, generate hormonal responses that include the release of estrogen.

This controlled release contributes to a hormonal balance that promotes both bone and cardiovascular health.

Promotion of Cardiovascular Function :

An Intrinsic Link with the Optimus4D System

The deep connection between our system and cardiovascular health lies where metabolic training stands as the architect of a vibrant and resilient heart life. Not a vague statement, but a dive into how this revolutionary system specifically addresses cardiac challenges through hormonal optimization.

The heart of the issue lies in hormonal balance, and the training system we employ at Optimus4D uniquely embraces this. As we explore the proper levels of different hormone levels , we understand how these are not only crucial for muscle health , but also for overall cardiovascular health.

Jaguar Beast's meticulously designed metabolic training routines not only influence hormonal levels, but act as a gatekeeper to optimal cardiovascular function. Reducing the risk of heart disease, this system stands as a proactive advocate for heart health.

So, get ready to explore how promoting cardiovascular function is not just a promise, but a commitment backed by science and realized through the system that Optimus4D employs. Your heart beats strongly not only from physical efforts, but from the knowledge that you are building a robust foundation for a thriving heart life.

Go ahead and discover the journey to long-lasting cardiovascular vitality with Optimus4D Metabolic Training!

Conclusions of this chapter

Integrating Hormonal Balance

The hormonal balance triggered by metabolic training represents a crucial component for overall health. Regular practice of this type of training not only positively impacts muscle development and fat burning, but also influences hormonal homeostasis, promoting a state of balance and well-being in the body. Some notable findings include:

1. Optimization of Anabolic Hormones : Metabolic training favors the release of anabolic hormones, such as growth hormone (GH), which plays fundamental roles in protein synthesis, muscle development and cell regeneration.

2. Stress and Cortisol Control: Regular practice of metabolic exercise contributes to stress management through the release of endorphins, counteracting the negative effects of cortisol. This helps maintain balanced cortisol levels, avoiding chronic elevations that can have adverse impacts on health.

3. Regulation of Insulin Sensitivity : Metabolic training improves insulin sensitivity, facilitating more efficient management of glucose in the body. This is crucial to prevent metabolic problems such as insulin resistance and type 2 diabetes.

4. Stability in Adrenaline and Norepinephrine Levels : I did not go into this and it is not a mistake that I mention it here now as an extra so that you keep it in mind that The metabolic response to these training involves the release of catecholamines such as adrenaline and norepinephrine. These hormones play a role in energy mobilization and the body's adaptation to physical exertion.

5. Improvement of Mood and Reduction of Psychological Stress : I was more extensive on this, he release of endorphins during metabolic exercise not only has analgesic effects, but also contributes to a general feeling of well-being and improved mood, counteracting psychological stress.

Together, these positive hormonal effects provide a solid foundation for holistic health. Metabolic workouts don't just focus on aesthetic or performance aspects, they address the interconnection between exercise, hormonal responses, and overall well-being. The key lies in consistency and tailoring these workouts to individual needs, providing a holistic approach to maintaining hormonal balance over time.

Chapter III

Exploring the Countless Benefits From the JaguarBeast Method

3.1 Effective Burning of Calories: Discovering Continuous Power

In this fascinating section, you will immerse yourself in the incredible reality of persistent calorie burning. Metabolic Training is not simply an exercise routine; It is an ongoing commitment to your physical well-being. Studies conducted by the University of Colorado (Smith et al., 2018) reveal the amazing ability of this approach to keep your metabolism active even after you have completed your training from 48 to 60 hours later. You will explore how this phenomenon translates not only into effective weight loss, but into the creation of an internal engine that drives long-term physical health.

3.2 Time Efficiency:

Deep Learning to Maximize Every Minute

Going into the heart of time efficiency, this section is a revelation about how Metabolic Training optimizes every moment of your session. Findings from McMaster University (Gillen et al., 2016) illuminate the effectiveness of shorter but intense sessions. You will learn to challenge traditional time conventions and get the most out of every minute of training. This section is your guide to redefining the relationship between time spent and results obtained, a paradigm shift that will set the tone for your physical transformation journey.

And in this section I am inspired to leave the field of science and training for a moment and leave you a more inspirational message, because I can help you get the most out of the time you spend training, but not the time you spend with the rest or When you decide to take part of that valuable time and invest it in your best version.

"Time is the fabric of our lives, a precious fabric that only we can embroider. Every moment is an opportunity, a blank canvas waiting to be filled with the colors of our dreams. Take advantage of every tick of the clock as a gift, a unique opportunity to create, grow and love. Do not underestimate the value of every second; it is the most valuable treasure we possess. May every beat of your heart remind you of the wonderful opportunity you have to live, learn and leave an indelible mark on the world. canvas of time."

3.3 Improved Stamina and Energy:

Exploring Unexplored Levels of Vitality

In this exploration of the unique combination of cardiovascular exercises combined with endurance and strength, you will discover how JaguarBeast Method Metabolic Training is not only a physical activity, but an elixir that nourishes endurance and energy.

Studies from Harvard University (Ratey, 2018) highlight how this approach has a profound impact on cognitive function and mental health. The vitality you gain from these sessions goes beyond mere physical activity; It is an awakening of your unexplored potential.

Be part of this reality where each heartbeat, each movement, propels you towards new levels of vitality, both in each training session and in your daily life.

3.4 Adaptability to Different Aptitudes:

Examining Custom Versatility

By thoroughly examining the intrinsic versatility of Metabolic Training, you will understand that this is not a one-size-fits-all approach. Studies from the Mayo Clinic (Swift et al., 2018) support the adaptability of this method for people of all fitness levels. Whether you're a beginner taking the first steps on your fitness journey or an experienced athlete, Metabolic Training is molded to your individual needs. You'll immerse yourself in the wealth of options and adjustments, discovering how each routine fits you, providing you with a personalized path to continuous improvement.

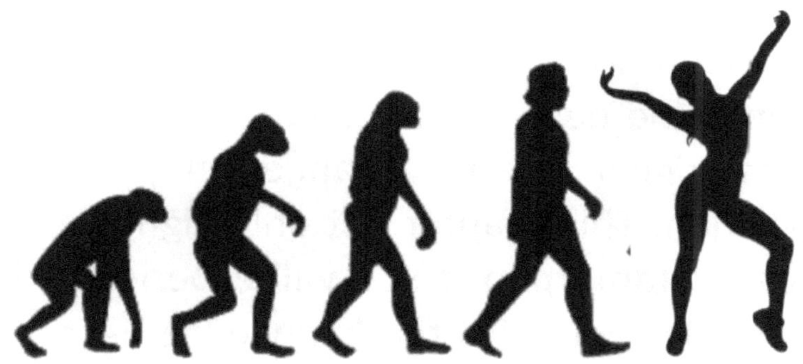

3. 5 Benefits for Mental Health:

Discovering the Mind-Body Symphony

In this deep dive into the science of holistic transformation, we go beyond simple weight loss and explore how Metabolic Training becomes a meticulous architect of body reshaping.

Detailed studies by the International Society of

Sports Nutrition (Helms et al., 2014) provide strong support for the idea that this approach not only targets fat loss, but also drives gains in lean muscle mass.

On this fascinating journey, you will not only observe how each exercise series contributes to a visible external transformation, but you will also delve into the deep understanding of how these routines trigger internal changes in your body composition. This chapter not only highlights the physical metamorphosis you will experience, but also provides you with the knowledge necessary to understand how each specific movement and exercise works synergistically to sculpt a healthier, more vital body.

Through the detailed lens of research and science, I lift the curtain a little to reveal to you the mysteries behind the holistic transformation that awaits you when you adopt Metabolic Training. It is not simply an exercise program; is a comprehensive strategy designed to optimize your body composition from the inside out, creating a sustainable and lasting change in your overall well-being.

You'll discover how each routine not only works your muscles, but also your mind, reducing stress, improving mood, and promoting overall mental health. When you introduce these sections you immerse yourself in the perfect harmony between body and mind, where each heartbeat and each breath contribute to your overall well-being and for this you do not need to wait long weeks or months because I dare to assure you based on the opinion of thousands of my students . that you will enjoy this benefit in the first week.

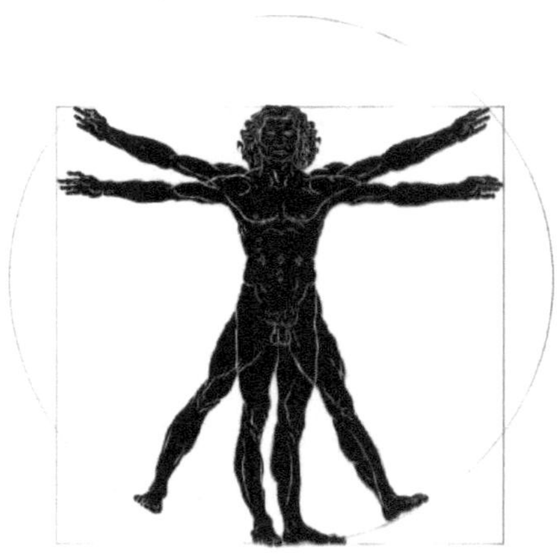

Conclusion Chapter 3: Setting the Groundwork for Lasting Transformation

By the conclusion of this extensive chapter, you will have explored the multiple layers of the benefits of Metabolic Training. Every word, every study, has been designed to give you a complete and rich view of how this approach goes beyond the expectations you would expect .

It is evident that it leads to persistent calorie burning , you have learned that the method helps you maximize every minute of your training, exploring the deepest levels of vitality, highlighting adaptability to different levels of fitness, revealing to you the holistic transformation of body composition, leading you to feel the symphony between mind and body. This chapter lays the foundation for your journey toward lasting and meaningful transformation.

Get ready for the next chapter, where you will continue exploring the wonders you can achieve with the Optimus4D system at the center and the Jaguar Beast Method in its Online version!

<u>Metabolic Program 4D</u>

CHAPTER IV

METABOLIC TRAINING PROGRAM

JAGUAR BEAST METHOD

Welcome to the heart of the Jaguar Beast Method of the Optimus4D system:

The Training Program designed with the commitment to bring you wherever you are, the benefits of this method that has been studied, organized and rigorously measured, tested on myself and on hundreds of my students, putting to the test what is indicated by the different studies that explain the magnificent results and benefits , adapting, adjusting and perfecting until you have what I offer you today as the "JaguarBeast" metabolic training.

In this chapter, I will provide you with a detailed exercise plan designed to maximize your results in record time. These routines can be done at home or anywhere with little space and equipment. Get ready to activate your body and accelerate your metabolism.

4.1 Principles of Metabolic Training

Before we dive into the routines, it is essential to understand the fundamental principles of Jaguar Beast Method Training. These routines focus on compound movements that work several muscle groups at once, but with a specific focus periodicity on each muscle group, for which I have based myself on a 3-day approach in which. The combination. Strategically, the time of performing the exercises is crucial to maximize the metabolic response to offer you time efficiency.

In the title of this book I specify 9 minutes. And this is because in that time you will have already activated the EPOC window* Which will make it possible for you to continue obtaining calorie burning results after 48 hours after exercise, understanding that you are performing the necessary intensity.

My workouts are based on completing 18 minutes, but you have to understand that, if you are starting out and your physical abilities do not allow you to complete this time, 9 minutes will be what you have to strive to complete to open this metabolic window and advance in your physical condition, your energy and your strength, until you complete the 18 minutes, if you wish. And reach the recommended maximum of 45 that we do in the tribe... (relative to the intensity of the day)

I have to be completely honest with you and that is that, experienced athletes, by being able to give one hundred percent of their capacity from the beginning, can open this metabolic window in just 4 minutes. In fact, it is used in Olympic programs by athletes. high performance, I make the reference in case you have come to think that perhaps this program is like a warm washcloth to get you through the problem, not at all!!! It's high-level, grounded training, so trust the process.

This above is what is known as the Tabata method and is perfect for specific moments, but not to provide you with long-term general health metabolic benefits. In fact, I recommend it and I provide you with demonstration videos so that you can do them at specific moments .

I have experienced it myself, Tabata at its highest level, but I do not work under these bases with my partners and students because I understand that it requires a greater capacity to control our condition and physical abilities and it is not that I question its possibilities or abilities in fact. I trust, I believe, and I assure my students that they will be able to feel like athletes, but there are certain thresholds that simply do not seem necessary to me.

In addition to the fact that we are not competitive athletes, although we could become one , we are not preparing for the Olympics.

So, as in general, the primary objective now is to maintain excellent physical shape, feel good, be proud of the results and our appearance, to manage to proudly go through the years and not be trampled by them. Like everything that involves your emotional sensations, which will lead you to a healthy mind, better relationships and better results in your daily life, as you may have heard philosophers say, Mens sana in corpore sana . And this is an absolute reality. Does your body influence the health of your mind? And your mind. It influences health. Of your body.

If you have not yet done any online, in-person training or the material that I offer you recorded and free on my YouTube channel, you have to know the following example is generic and does not capture the essence of the intuitive training that we offer you in any of its formats, no. However, in addition to all of the above, you also have the complete "JaguarBeast" training program available in downloadable format with a lifetime membership . I will leave you a link to what I detail under this training example.

4.2 Exemplified Routine

Warm up (5 minutes)

- Rope Jumping: 2 minutes

- Activate your cardiovascular system and improve circulation.

- Arm and Leg Rotation: 2 minutes

- Increases mobility and prepares joints for exercise.

- Squats with Rotation: 1 minute

- Combine leg and trunk movements to involve different muscle groups.

Development (15 minutes)

This routine focuses on full-body exercises to maximize calorie burn and improve overall strength.

1. Bodyweight Squats

- Keep your feet shoulder-width apart, slowly lower yourself down and return to the starting position.

- Repetitions: 15-20.

Push-ups

- Place your hands just outside shoulder width, lower your body and return to the starting position.

- Repetitions: 10-15.

3. Lunges (3 minutes)

- Take a step forward, lower your hips and repeat with the other leg.

- Repetitions: 12-16.

4. Jaguar Iron

- Hold a plank position with your body in a straight line from head to heels and start the movement that you will see in the video

5. Burpees

- **Combines a squat, a push-up and a vertical jump in one fluid movement.**

- **Repetitions: 10-12.**

The objective is to perform these exercises, rest for about 25 seconds between them and start again from 1 to 5 a total of 4 times maximum and minimum 2 times.

Stretch and cool down (5 minutes)

- Dynamic Stretches (2 minutes)

- Perform dynamic stretches to relax the worked muscles.

- Deep Breathing and Relaxation (3 minutes)

- Give your body time to recover and reduce your heart rate.

Come in, observe and get ready to do a routine with me, I leave you the link to a training session, and you can also request a free week of training with me as your personal trainer.

Targeted training 18Minutes keep time with me

You have the links and QR codes in the following information

Let's train together

Contact me __

4.3 Recommended Equipment

Adjustable dumbbells To add resistance to exercises. (This does not necessarily have to be weights as such, you can use bottles with sand, water or any object that weighs and you can hold comfortably) Although I recommend weights for their comfort

Resistance band Ideal for strengthening exercises, it can make it much easier for you to go with bottles and weights because its use can be configured in many ways.

Mat: Although it seems the most dispensable, it is important when you lie down or place your hands and knees in contact with the ground, because otherwise you will not be able to concentrate on the exercise thinking about what the support is hurting you.

Click and QR interactive actions

video example that I mentioned or if you have a physical copy you can scan the QR that will take you to the example videos where you can see the detailed movements to guarantee precise and safe execution.

Refer to these images while you train to maximize the benefits and reduce the risk of injury.

In the previous lines in the exercises you have an example of this and within the Jaguar Beast program you will have it in mind in each plan that I offer you.

Conclusion of Chapter 4

This Training Program considered Express , of the JaguarBeast Method , named for its possibilities of obtaining important benefits by completing the first 9 minutes of the program, offers you the opportunity to transform your body in just a few minutes a day and this is literal .

Remember to adapt routines according to your fitness level and listen to your body. Get ready to experience the efficiency and effectiveness of a workout designed to fit perfectly into your busy lifestyle!

CHAPTER V

Tips for Integration

JaguarBeast in the Daily Routine

Fitting training into a busy day may seem like a monumental challenge, but with the right strategies, it's possible to create healthy habits that fit seamlessly into your daily routine. In this chapter, we'll explore practical and effective tips for integrating Jaguar Beast Method training routines into your everyday life, addressing time management and creating lasting habits.

5.1 Establish Clear and Realistic Goals

Before embarking on your training journey, set clear and achievable goals. Break your goals down into smaller, more specific goals, which will make it easier to plan your daily routine.

5.2 Create a Fixed Training Schedule

Assign a specific time for your workout and treat

it like any other important appointment. This creates consistency and makes it easier to incorporate exercise into your daily routine.

5.3 Short and Effective Training Sessions

Make the most of the time available. Jaguar Beast Method training sessions are short but effective. Schedule your sessions at strategic times, such as in the morning before work or during lunch, in the case of training on your own, if you have the opportunity to be part of The VIP Tribe, congratulations, your progress is assured, being independent with our method as well. , but you have to have more will, trust yourself.

5.4 Integrate Training into Daily Activities

Look for opportunities to incorporate movement into your day. Take the stairs instead of the elevator, park farther away to walk more, or do brief stretches during breaks at work.

5.5 Focus on Consistency over Intensity

Prioritize consistency instead of intensity. Regular sessions, even if they are shorter, are preferable to sporadic and exhausting efforts.

That is why I recommend that even just reaching the 9-minute mark is 100% success.

5.6 Make Training a Priority

Recognize the importance of your health and well-being. By making training a priority, you commit to improving your quality of life in the long term.

5.7 Involve a Training Partner

Training with a partner not only makes exercise more fun, but also provides mutual accountability.

This great advantage is what you can obtain by being part of the tribe, whether online or in person, because you will connect at specific times, you will be in your own group and you will create the commitment to train with them.

Plan sessions with friends or family to make training a social activity.

5.8 Prepare Equipment in Advance

Reduce barriers to entry by preparing your equipment in advance. Leave your workout clothes ready the night before and place any necessary equipment in an accessible location.

5.9 Celebrate Small Accomplishments

Recognize and celebrate every achievement, no matter how small it may seem . This reinforces the positive mindset and motivates you to keep going.

5.10 Adapt to Changes in Routine

Life is full of changes, and your routine may be affected. Learn to adapt and find creative ways to keep exercise in your life, even in the midst of challenges.

Conclusion of Chapter V

Successfully integrating training into your daily routine not only improves your physical health, but also contributes to greater mental clarity and emotional resilience. Follow these practical tips and watch the Jaguar Beast Method become a vital and sustainable part of your busy lifestyle.

Get ready to discover how small changes can have a significant impact on your overall well-being!

Optimus4D Group

SUCCESS TESTIMONIALS
IN THE OPTIMUS4D TRIBE

Nothing tells the narrative of victory in a training program better than the authentic experiences of those who have undergone an extraordinary transformation. In this chapter, we will enthusiastically share dozens of inspiring testimonies from busy individuals, entrepreneurs, fathers, mothers who have successfully incorporated the authentic Training Method, together with the Optimus4D Tribe, into their lives. These stories serve as a testament that positive change can be achieved even in the midst of busy schedules.

It won't take long for you to know many of these people and their stories personally and be part of them too, because if you become an Optimus4D person with all your four "Ds"

DESIRE – DECISION – DETERMINATION AND DISCIPLINE

I don't assure you that it will be successful,

I GUARANTEE YOU!!!

Carla, 35 years old, Project Manager

"With my busy schedule, I always thought exercise was out of my reach. But thanks to one day accepting Will's challenge to connect to an Optimus4D Tribe workout, now my training sessions are my sanctuary, my sacred time to "recharge myself and face the day with more energy."

Javier, 42 years old, Businessman

"As an entrepreneur, I was always stressed and had no time for the gym. But the effective JaguarBeast Method from my now also Optimus4D Tribe fit perfectly into my lifestyle. After weeks, I not only lost weight, but also noticed a significant improvement in my focus and productivity.

Marta, 38 years old, Full-Time Mother

"Raising three children is exhausting, but with the Optimus4D Tribe, I discovered that even 15 minutes a day can make a big difference. Now, I have more energy to play with my children and keep up with their activities."

Andrés, 45 years old, Health Professional

"As a doctor, my schedule is unpredictable. Thanks to the ingenious JaguarBeast Method, I can stay in shape without compromising my attention to patients. This method is my ally for comprehensive well-being, even in free time in the clinic I can take advantage and train."

Laura, 37 years old, Graduate Student

"Studies often consume my time, but the efficient JaguarBeast Method allowed me to incorporate exercise without affecting my academic responsibilities. I feel more focused and balanced." Plus, it's my escape valve when exams overwhelm me.

Roberto, 40 years old, Frequent Traveler for Work

"Constant travel made maintaining an exercise routine difficult. But Optimus4D's adaptable

JaguarBeast Method is my constant travel companion, giving me the flexibility I need to stay fit anywhere in the world."

Ana, 36 years old, Entrepreneur

"As an entrepreneur, I am always on the go. And I couldn't find a way to go to a gym and at home it seemed like I was wasting time, but with the Optimus4D Tribe it fits my dynamic lifestyle and is also effective. It has transformed my energy and resilience, allowing me to face each challenge with confidence."

Isabel, 41 years old, Creative FreeLancer

"Creativity often comes with long hours of work. Incorporating the effective Jaguar Beast Method and now being part of the Optimus4D Tribe not only helped me stay fit, but also improved my mental clarity and creative ability."

Pedro, 39 years old, Shift Worker

"Working rotating shifts made it difficult to maintain a consistent routine. But with the versatile JaguarBeast Method, I can train at any time of the day, adapting to my variable schedule. But whenever it coincides I definitely connect to direct training."

Don't forget to listen to these testimonies from people like you and me, who one day decided to bet on themselves and leave aside fears, excuses and "esques"

Scan or Click if you have the E-book version

JaguarBeast

ADDITIONAL RESOURCES

In this sixth chapter, you will find a wealth of additional resources supported by the exceptional Optimus4D Tribe and the effective JaguarBeast Method, designed to enrich your training experience.

On my YouTube about training, you can find and support different routines in which I share and perform the complete training so you can follow me

Immerse yourself in a complete library of demo videos from the Optimus4D Tribe. Discover the precise form of each JaguarBeast Method exercise, ensuring effective and safe execution.

Access the You Tube channel HERE

And if this technology fails you can search:

Will Optimus4D
@willcastillooptimus4d79

My 3 BestSeller book **"Jaguar Mindset and Strength"** has helped many to unleash their maximum potential and make training a lasting habit, knowing the mental patterns behind our failure in this area despite knowing its importance.

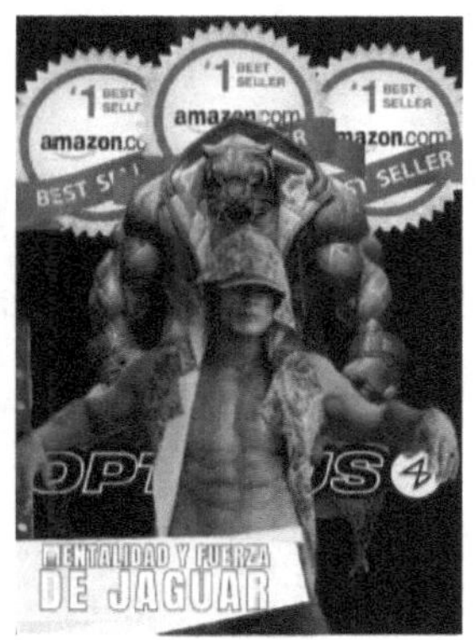

In it you will find knowledge unknown to 90% of people who fail in their attempt to carry out activities that contribute to the care of their health, you will not find routines, you will not find diets, you will find the definitive solution to whatever decision you make in In this area you will finally be able to be constant, be successful and never give up again...

Discover the secret of the mental patterns of your generation in this book, I assure you you will be surprised by everything you will discover, and in the same way you will also know more about my life story.

Jaguar Mentality and Strength book on Amazon and the best bookstores **You can Click on this line or go to the Amazon search engine**

JaguarBeast

@OPTIMUS_4D

Follow us on Instagram and be inspired by each story and publication where you can see people focused on achieving their best version just like you, achieving consistency more easily

Instagram:_optimus4D Click HERE

This reference is very important, because, without a doubt, I represent a before and after in the health of my family. The best discovery I have made and believe me when I tell you that I have done a lot of research before being able to speak with this confidence and security, about this device, in addition to the years that I have already used it. Not to mention that the greatest athletes in the world use it... I hope you tell me what you think

Only 3 minutes separate you from a great discovery

Click here

Access with

Password:

tribukangen

JaguarBeast

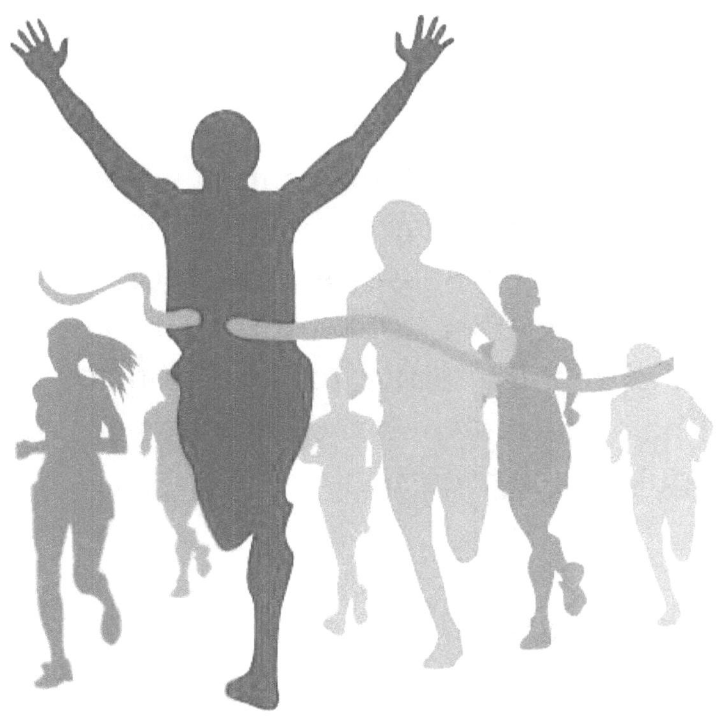

Ferocities Jaguar, you are at the goal of this book, that already says a lot about your dedication and commitment to finishing something when you set your mind to it, I hope to stay in touch with you and continue growing together, on the path to your best version.

JaguarBeast

Assuming Lasting Transformation

With the Optimus4D Tribe

WHY is it for you? "JaguarBeast Metabolic Training" is not just an exercise program; is an open door to total transformation supported by the exceptional Optimus4D Tribe and their innovative JaguarBeast Method. More than just a routine book, this book represents an exciting, personalized invitation to take control of your well-being, even when the demands of your busy schedule reach their peak.

In these pages, you've discovered a wealth of knowledge backed by science, but the real magic lies in putting these principles into practice. Here lies the key: applying the JaguarBeast Method not only as a series of exercises, but as a daily commitment to yourself. Because you are here and because you are looking for excellent results, the door is open, but my recommendation goes further.

Because Joining the Optimus4D Tribe is the next logical step in your transformation journey. Why face the challenge alone? when you can count on the guidance, support and motivation of real professionals in real time. The Optimus4D Tribe is not just a community; It is a support system that will surround you with people who share your goals, your struggles and your triumphs.

Imagine having access to certified trainers who will guide you through each session, adjust your exercises to your specific needs, and provide that extra boost when motivation flags. With the Tribe, every achievement is celebrated collectively, and every challenge is met with the support of a community that understands your journey.

This book is the beginning, but the Optimus4D Tribe is the natural continuation of your path to an active and healthy lifestyle. Personalized guidance, real-time interactions, and ongoing support will take you beyond what you could achieve on your own.

Click here to see all the communication options

Why wait?...

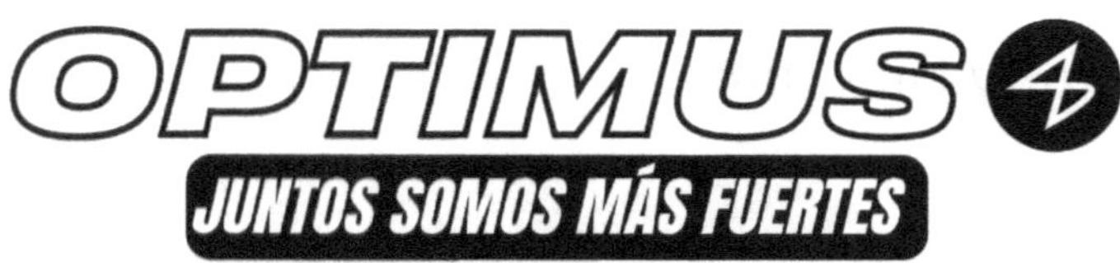

The Best Training System

JaguarBeast

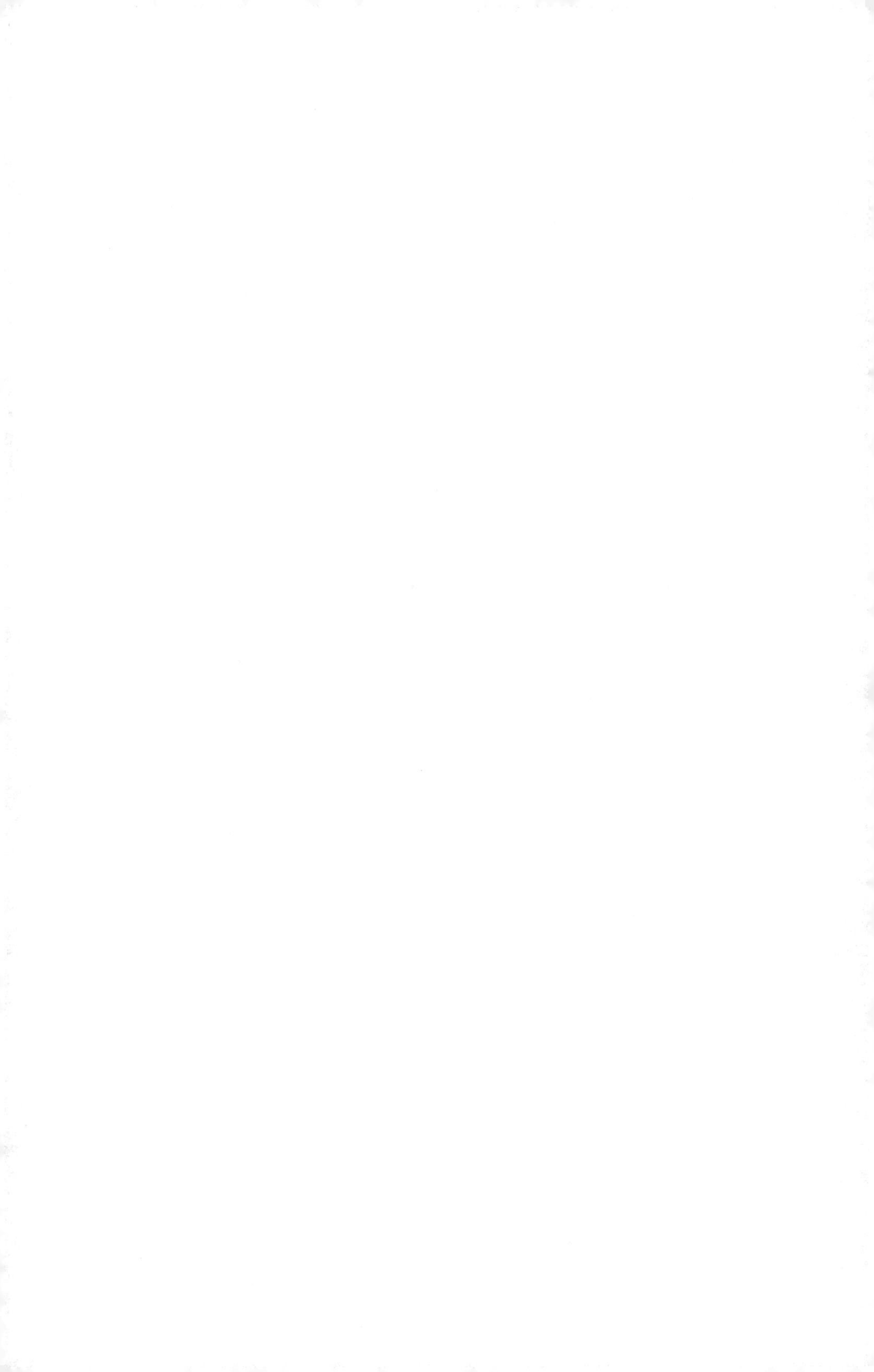

Building The life you want Everyday

Blueprint for successful living

By Gladys M.Bell

Table of content

Chapter 1: Defining Your Vision

The Power of Vision
In the hustle and bustle of our daily lives,
it's easy to lose sight of our deepest desires
and dreams. We become entangled in the
routines, obligations, and distractions that
life throws our way. Yet, within each of us
lies the capacity to dream, to aspire, and to
envision a future that resonates with our
truest selves. This is the essence of vision.
Vision is the compass that guides your
choices, the lighthouse in the stormy sea of
uncertainty. It provides clarity amidst chaos,
purpose amidst confusion, and motivation
amidst challenges. Your vision is uniquely
yours, and it serves as the North Star of your
life's journey.
Consider the story of Sarah, a young woman
who dreamed of opening a community
center in her underserved neighborhood.

Her vision was a place where children could receive academic support, families could access resources, and the community could come together to thrive. With this vision in mind, Sarah not only completed her education but also rallied support from local leaders, secured funding, and ultimately turned her dream into a reality. Sarah's vision was the driving force behind her actions, pushing her forward even when the path seemed daunting.

Clarifying Your Goals

Once you've embraced the significance of having a vision, the next step is to transform that vision into tangible goals. Goals are the bridge between your dreams and your reality. They break down the vastness of your vision into manageable, actionable steps.

Think of your vision as a grand tapestry with each thread representing a goal. These goals are Specific, Measurable, Achievable, Relevant, and Time-bound (SMART). They provide structure and direction to your journey. Instead of saying, "I want to be financially secure," you might set a SMART goal such as "I will save $10,000 in the next 12 months."

By setting such clear and concrete objectives, you gain a roadmap for progress. Each goal achieved is like a milestone on your path to building the life you want, bringing you closer to the grand tapestry of your vision.

Exploring Your Passions

Your vision isn't just about accomplishing tasks; it's about creating a life that resonates with your passions and values. Your passions are the colors that infuse vibrancy into your vision.

Consider the story of John, an engineer who felt unfulfilled in his career. He discovered his passion for teaching and mentoring young minds. By aligning his goals with his newfound passion, John transitioned into an educational role, ultimately becoming an influential educator who touched the lives of countless students.

Take the time to explore your own passions
and interests. What activities make your
heart sing? What could you do for hours
without feeling drained? Aligning your goals
with your passions can turn the pursuit of
your vision into an exciting and purposeful
journey.

Visualization Techniques

Visualization is a powerful tool that
transforms abstract ideas into concrete
realities. It's like sketching the blueprint of
your dream life before you start building.
Through visualization, you create a mental
movie of your desired future, complete with
sights, sounds, and emotions.

Imagine, for a moment, that your vision is to
become a successful writer. Close your eyes
and picture yourself sitting at your dream
writing desk, the soft glow of a lamp
illuminating your words. Feel the weight of
your book in your hands as you hold it for
the first time. This mental image becomes a
source of motivation, a reminder of your
aspirations, and a guide for your actions

Chapter 2 Setting Meaningful Goals

Setting goals is more than just listing desires; it's about crafting a roadmap to your future. To do this effectively, you need the SMART framework. Each element of SMART—Specific, Measurable, Achievable, Relevant, and Time-bound—is like a pillar, supporting the structure of your goals.
Specific: Your goals should be clear and precise. Vague goals like "I want to be successful" lack direction. Instead, a specific goal would be "I want to start my own business in the next year."
Measurable: Measuring progress keeps you accountable and motivated. When you can track your advancement, you gain a sense of achievement. For example, "I will save $5,000 by the end of this year" is measurable.
Achievable: While aiming high is commendable, setting realistic goals is essential. Aiming for the stars is inspiring, but setting impossible goals can lead to

frustration. Make sure your goals are attainable within your current circumstances.

Relevant: Goals should align with your vision. Ask yourself if a particular goal serves your ultimate purpose. If it doesn't, reconsider or adjust it. Your goals should be relevant to your life's direction.

Time-bound: Set a deadline for each goal. A time frame provides urgency and prevents procrastination. Without a deadline, goals can linger indefinitely. "I will complete a professional certification in six months" is time-bound.

Breaking Down Your Vision

Imagine your vision as a grand puzzle, and each goal as a piece that fits together to form the complete picture. Breaking down your vision into smaller, manageable goals is like assembling the puzzle, piece by piece. This process ensures you always know the next step to take.

Suppose your vision is to lead a healthier lifestyle. Break it down into smaller goals, such as "Exercise for 30 minutes every day," "Cook healthy meals four times a week," or "Lose 10 pounds in three months." These smaller goals become milestones, guiding your journey towards your vision.

Short-Term vs. Long-Term Goals

Balance is key when setting goals. Short-term goals offer quick wins, providing a sense of accomplishment and motivation. They are the daily and weekly tasks that keep you on track. Long-term goals, on the other hand, give you a sense of purpose and direction, often requiring more time and effort to achieve.

Consider the example of writing a book. Your short-term goals might include writing a certain number of pages each day or week, while your long-term goal is completing the entire manuscript. This balance between short and long-term goals ensures you stay motivated and focused on the bigger picture.
.

Staying Motivated

Goal setting is a journey, not a destination. Along the way, you'll encounter challenges, distractions, and moments of doubt. That's where motivation comes into play.
Celebrating Small Wins: Acknowledge and celebrate your achievements, even the small ones. Each step forward is progress.
Visualization: Picture yourself achieving your goals and living your vision. Visualization fuels your motivation and keeps your eyes on the prize.
Inspiration from Others: Seek inspiration from individuals who've achieved similar goals. Their stories remind you that success is possible, and they can offer valuable insights.
Accountability and Tracking Progress: Share your goals with someone you trust, whether it's a mentor, friend, or family member. This creates a sense of accountability.
Additionally, keep a journal to track your progress, providing evidence of your journey.
Adapting to Changing Circumstances

Life is unpredictable. Goals set today might need adjustment tomorrow. That's okay. Flexibility and adaptability are key to successful goal setting. If circumstances change or you discover a new direction, don't hesitate to revise your goals. It's not a failure; it's a sign of growth and awareness

Chapter 3 Overcoming obstacles

Beating deterrents and making progress requires you to make a move. You won't be aware on the off chance that it's a smart activity until you've wandered down the path of your choice. There was something wrong with it, so don't permit yourself to get enveloped with it. Simply grin to yourself and say, "OK, I just learned another way to avoid something," and continue on. Every disappointment and resulting achievement began with making do, executing, adjusting, and surviving. "Hindrances are there to stop the others who don't have the mental fortitude or the ability to make do around them." The way to build a triumphant outlook is to have a propensity for asking yourself, "Is there a superior method for doing this?" Looking for a superior way, regardless of what challenge you face, will lead you to overcome hindrances and make progress. Try not to stand by to pose this inquiry when you're trapped in a corner. Ask it whenever, during your excursion, you stumble into somebody going with a choice. This could be in a news story, a magazine, a book, the homeroom, on a games field, or on the Web. The fact of the matter is that building a triumphant outlook happens at the present time, not right when you want it. Like anything you practice, the more you do it, the better you'll get. Heaps of individuals will think of a superior method for following through with something, but what will isolate you from every other person is that you will make a move on your thoughts. At the point when a snag divides you and your objective, grin with certainty and realize that the obstruction is there to stop the others who don't have the boldness or the readiness to make do around it. Seven Methods for Overcoming Obstructions and Making Progress Since we have a comprehension of the overall standards for picking the right attitude and making objectively driven moves to execute your thoughts and pursue your fantasies, we should survey particular ways of conquering impediments and making progress.

1. Have faith in yourself. Having a positive, killer instinct is fundamental when confronting hindrances and difficulties. Having confidence in yourself implies accepting that you are fit to accomplish your objectives, regardless of how large or small they might be. Before you can accomplish anything, you should initially accept. It's a significant message, yet it's not quite as basic as some would tell you: "I should simply accept, and I can accomplish anything I need." Obviously, you don't know—you feel somewhat skeptical. I know precisely the way that you feel. I was a youngster with asthma whose specialist said I ought to figure out how to play chess, and I was unable to try and play checkers well enough. Later on, as a business visionary, I learned 1,000,000, 400, or 75 thousand bucks worth of ways not to send off an item; what's more, a portion of my financial backers let me know the time had come to

quit humiliating myself and go find a new line of work. To beat obstructions and at last make progress, I needed to track down my motivation to accept.

2. Remain positive and hopeful: Definitely, there will be times when you stagger and face hindrances on the way to accomplishing your objectives. In those minutes, keeping a positive, hopeful standpoint and seeing every snag as a chance for growth is significant. The stunt is isolating the convictions that assist you from those that obstruct you. Also, making a move is a persistent activity, which is the immediate consequence of your convictions. You don't shed 25 pounds in a day, and you might have neglected to support persevering activity previously. The key is to perceive and zero in on the convictions that will assist you with achieving the objective you've picked. It's not exactly simple or easy; in any case, each time I accepted that I was unable to follow through with

something, I was correct. In any case, it was simply because I hadn't made a move!

3. Put forth objectives and work towards them: As opposed to just permitting hindrances and misfortunes to crash you, set objectives for yourself and work consistently towards accomplishing them. This will assist with keeping you focused on your ultimate objective, even despite misfortune. In the first place, you perceive motivation to accept, and that will come from the little triumphs in your day-to-day existence. Each time I accepted that I could follow through with something, I gained ground toward my course. Some of the time it didn't feel like advancement, as I just educated myself on a couple of ways to avoid something; however, it actually advanced in light of the fact that I didn't quit any pretense of accepting that I could make it happen! Rather than zeroing in on the pile of obstructions, significantly impact your viewpoint by utilizing perception, which includes envisioning yourself effectively

accomplishing your objectives and conquering the difficulties that you face. By envisioning achievement routinely, you can support your certainty and increase your odds of coming out on top, in actuality.

4. Continue on through difficult stretches: What you accept concludes what you should or shouldn't do! The key is tied in with imparting propensities that assist you in prevailing at the things you have some control over. You have no control over what others say, do, think, or feel; in any case, you have some control over how you will deal with things you have zero control over. You have some control over the course you take, and in particular, you have some control over your activities and your capacity to accept. Reevaluate misfortunes as growth opportunities. At the point when you experience impediments or misfortunes, search for the illustrations you can gain from them. Reexamining assists with moving your concentration away from pessimistic considerations or feelings. This

will assist you in becoming an individual
and drive you forward on your journey to
progress.

5. Make a move and don't delay:
Achievement comes from building
propensities that empower you to make the
right moves toward satisfying your fantasy. I
wasn't the smartest understudy in school,
nor was I the best competitor; hell, I wasn't
even the best Naval Force SEAL. However, I
made it my objective to be awesome at never
surrendering—at thinking ambitiously and
being actually responsible for making my
fantasies work out. Rather than abstaining
from provocations and putting off making a
move to tackle issues, embrace each issue by
saying, "Alright. Where's the open door?"
The issue will make me more grounded.
Separate bigger objectives into more
modest, more sensible advances. This
assists us with setting more sensible
assumptions, yet additionally gives us a
reasonable guide for accomplishing our
targets. By handling each little part in turn,

we can try not to feel overpowered and gain ground towards our objective.

6. Be ready and consistently learn: Being arranged means thinking about everything that can turn out badly and then concocting an emergency course of action. Some refer to this as "out-of-the-container" thinking; however, I call it three-dimensional preparation. Consider taking a gander at an arrangement from each point, where you need to go, yet in addition to the things that could adjust your direction, and plan how to manage them. You intend to set yourself up for the unforeseen. To get ready, one must initially design. The more your arrangement, the more you can get ready; the more you set up, the greater your odds of coming out on top. Some express, "Inability to design is anticipating disappointment." I say, "Embrace disappointment as a method for learning." Disappointment makes you more brilliant; it gives you responses and empowers you to turn out to be better. Try not to go for the

gold; when you do come up short, gain from it.

7. Help other people and offer in return: Encircle yourself with strong individuals. Having areas of strength for an organization can be basic in assisting you with defeating impediments and making progress. In anything critical that I've achieved, from driving three Naval Force SEAL detachments to running a quickly developing startup, I expected to collaborate with others who were perfect at the things I wasn't perfect at. Contacting companions, relatives, or other believed consultants can furnish you with important exhortations and support as you work through testing times. Besides the fact that we benefit straightforwardly from having areas of strength for an organization, when we begin serving and having an effect on others, we're not pondering our own predicament any longer. We're pondering lifting others up, being worth it to other people, and keeping away from the snares of self-indulgence and

situational sorrow, which are extremely ordinary responses. Beating Snags and Making Progress Means to Carry Out, Adjust, and Survive: Execute an activity, adjust to the outcome, and rehash until you've defeated the snag. Resemble a stream and track down your way finished, under, around, or through—consistently continue on and don't quit streaming. Your prosperity will come from your capacity to continue on. Achievement is feasible assuming that you have the right mentality and will try sincerely to overcome impediments. These seven hints will assist in showing you the way to progress. Simply make sure to never abandon your fantasies, and the sky is the limit! Look at our Assets and Courses segments for more data on conquering hindrances, fostering your flexibility, further developing your general prosperity, and arriving at your maximum capacity. Also, remember to pursue our free month-to-month bulletin to get standard

tips, motivation, and guidance conveyed
directly to your inbox.

Chapter 4 Build a support system

It takes a town to bring up a youngster. It takes a town to endure school. It takes a town to begin another business. It takes a town to move into another area. It takes a town to conquer tension, sadness, or dependence. It takes a town to endure separation. It takes a town to lament a misfortune. It takes a town to endure a pandemic. Anything that you are carrying on with throughout everyday life, positive or negative, takes a town. Since you are not intended to go through it alone, During positive times, individuals around you enrich the positive minutes. Their presence, fervor, and joy add real meaning. Since we are wired for social association, it may seem OK that our euphoria is increased when we share it with those we love. Consider the time you landed that position; who did you call to share the news? Consider the time you got your most memorable check; who did you take out for lunch? Consider the time you had a break from work; who did you enjoy it with? We normally go to those we love to share the positive moments in our lives. We know that those in our emotionally supportive network not only know the battle we have gone through to arrive at this achievement, yet they likewise share our satisfaction and fervor. We realize that they are as glad for us as we are for ourselves. We get a feeling of fulfillment and satisfaction when we can impart our euphoria to everyone around us. Positive social help and social collaboration assist us in carrying on with our lives all the more completely. Conversely, the emotionally supportive network turns into the magic that binds it when we are going through difficult situations. They become our beacon that provides us with guidance. With such a long way to go in 2020, we have had a lot of motivations to require our emotionally supportive network. The occasions of this current year have been more seriously debilitating, exhausting, and testing than any time in recent memory. In addition to the fact that we confronted kinds of stress that we had no past openness or involvement in, the force of the sensations of tension, outrage, and misfortune arrived at new levels. The majority of us felt like none of the apparatuses in our tool compartment were useful, powerful, or solid. We felt like helpless souls most days. While managing all the obscure and vulnerable things around us, we can encounter more pressure, nervousness, and sadness. We can feel lacking and frail when tackling our concerns. Extreme feelings adjust our sense of trust in ourselves. Extreme feelings change our discernments, prompting more slanted and pessimistic ends. The truth of the matter is that at the point at which our feelings are high, our discernment is low. At the point when we become involved with our negative reasoning, an emotionally supportive network can be a solid sounding board for us. Individuals in our emotionally supportive network can assist us with thoroughly considering things all the more soundly, to issue tackle all the more really, and to completely remain present in our lives more. Our emotionally supportive network is a solid and compelling asset that can help us over the course of dim times. 3 Advantages Areas of Strength for a Solid Emotionally Supportive Network: There are numerous ways we can have a positive and emotionally supportive network in our lives. It very well may be through family, companions, neighbors, parent gatherings, coaches, and partners. A portion of those individuals might have been in our lives since we were small children, while others might turn out to be in our lives briefly as we change through various sections of our lives. You might have had an extraordinary teacher or a flatmate in school who helped you through the yearning to go home or the difficulties of the scholarly world. You might have had companions from secondary school who were at your wedding. You might have new companions as you branch out into being a parent. Regardless of how long this strong figure has been in your emotionally supportive network and what brought them into your life, there are not many widespread advantages to having them in your day-to-day existence. An emotionally supportive network can give insight and direction. During troublesome times, we frequently feel stuck. You feel deadened and befuddled, and you don't see any good reason to have hope. It gets hard to conclude what is awesome after the next stage, so you freeze and sit idle. A strong and soundly encouraging group of people can be the solid individuals in your life that assist you with getting unstuck. These individuals in your circle utilize their own background, schooling, and preparation to impart to you to track down arrangements and survival techniques for your concern. Emotionally supportive networks like a mentor, teacher, or tutor can furnish you with the direction you want as you work on your fantasies. It can have assets that will instruct and educate you regarding better approaches to taking care of your concerns. The insight of people around you takes a portion of the strain off your shoulders. At the point when you are encircled by those that lift you up, you draw nearer to your most elevated and most genuine potential. Your emotionally supportive network can play a significant role in your own and proficient turn of events. An emotionally supportive network can give strength and trust. During an upsetting time, self-uncertainty can get comfortable, leaving you feeling unreliable and deficient. You begin to lose trust in yourself. You begin to second-guess yourself, your capacities, and your abilities. You get found out in an endless loop among uncertainty and self-analysis. You begin to see all that is absent, rather than all that you have. You begin to see each of your inadequacies rather than every one of your assets. A decent, emotionally supportive network can be your cradle against those difficult stretches. Having everyone around you who puts stock in you and supports you can give you the certainty to continue to go. They help you remember your assets and power so you can refocus. You begin to benefit from their inspiration and begin to reduce most, if not all, connections with uncertainty and frailty. Positive individuals around you can impart trust in you. An emotionally supportive network can give understanding and sympathy. There will be minutes where arrangements aren't promptly accessible. There will be times when you have done all you can that is within your control. There isn't anything you can accomplish more of. You have no control over the result. In those minutes, you really want association and friendship. Your emotionally supportive network can offer basic encouragement through compassion, understanding, and tolerance. On occasion, all you want is for somebody to accompany you at that time. Not to offer counsel or arrangement, not to offer ameliorating words like "being OK is all going," be that as it may, somebody who sits with you since you needn't bother with being distant from everyone else. Brene Brown is cited as saying that sympathy is tied in with having the option to sit in obscurity with others rather than turning on the light. At times we simply believe a shoulder should cry on, somebody who comprehends what we are going through and will sit with us in it. Do whatever it takes not to transform it; make an effort not to let us know that being alright, however, basically being at the time with us is going. Ways of building major areas of strength for a framework: Now that you have taken advantage of the advantages of having an emotionally supportive network in your life, both for the positive and the pessimistic moments, the time has come to get to work. The truth of the matter is that to fabricate strong, sound areas of strength for a network, you want to follow some activity steps. Distinguish Your Necessities: Having major areas of strength for your emotionally supportive network begins with you! For your emotionally supportive network to work for you, it must match your exceptional requirements, objectives, qualities, and shortcomings. You can ask yourself inquiries, for example, "What am I chipping away at the present moment?" and "What are my objectives, dreams, or vision?" "Where might I want to see myself by and by, or expertly, in a half year or one year from this point?" to recognize your requirements. To assist you with recognizing the help you want, you can ask yourself, "Where do I stall out?" "What do I want assistance with?" At the point when you recognize your requirements and objectives for yourself, you have clarity on where you are and where you need to go. This guide can more readily assist with distinguishing who in your life can uphold you on this excursion. At the point when you recognize your assets and shortcomings, you additionally have clarity around what others can propose for you with regards to your shortcomings and how others can uphold you with regards to your assets. This kind of purposefulness will bring more extravagance and satisfaction to the relationship. At the point when you distinguish how people around you best help and assist you, you can be better at valuing them. It can get more straightforward to show appreciation to everyone around us. The truth of the matter is that we go through numerous occasions and difficulties. We can't expect not many individuals in our emotionally supportive network to be accessible and prepared to help us for every one of them. At the point when you separate it and distinguish what your necessities are in a given circumstance and afterward have the option to recognize who you can connect with in this specific circumstance, not exclusively will the emotionally supportive network be successful in aiding you, but you will likewise feel satisfied and very much upheld. Connect and request help: Commonly, when we are amidst difficult stretches, we naturally think we are distant from everyone else in them. We ruminate on why it worked out and how we might have kept away from it, as though terrible things aren't intended to occur. The more we assume we are distant from everyone else in our torment, the harder it gets. We segregate ourselves rather than connecting. We will quite often fail to remember that we don't need to experience peace. Since the emotionally supportive network can be the wellbeing net that can direct us through the difficult stretches, So what prevents you from connecting and requesting help? All things considered, what benefit is an emotionally supportive network in the event that you are excessively timid or reluctant to utilize it? Frequently, we think back and wish we had relied on our emotionally supportive network prior to or on a more regular basis. You never hear somebody say, "I lament that I depended on my emotionally supportive network." What disrupts everything about requesting help? Normally, pessimistic sentiments play a part in evading requesting help. Sentiments like shame or pride hinder connecting. On the off chance that you have dread of being defenseless, you are bound to keep things inside. There can likewise be contorted discernments around the significance of requesting help. You might have come to accept that requesting help is an indication of a shortcoming. You imagine that doing it all alone is a greater accomplishment than allowing others to help. These kinds of nonsensical and pointless contemplations prevent you from requesting help. To contact your encouraging group of people, you would have to recognize any restricting convictions and reexamine them, so it gets simpler for you to request help. It can likewise be useful to speak with everyone around you about any difficulties you have with requesting help. This way, when you really do connect and request help, they know how hard it very well may be for you to be defenseless and make a point to answer you rapidly and straightforwardly. One final thing to consider while chipping away at connecting and requesting help is to realize that nobody can guess what you might be thinking. Nobody can know when you really want assistance or what sort of assistance you require. Thus, when you are connecting with somebody you trust, you should convey immovably, straightforwardly, and clearly. You should be explicit about when you really want assistance from them. Is it that second that you request help? Or, on the other hand, is it in a couple of days? Be likewise unambiguous about the means they can take to help you. Is there a particular errand they can take on or a particular expertise they can educate you on? The more open and informative you are about your necessities, the more certain it is for you to get the sort of help you really want. Give an encouraging group of people Consent to Keep You Responsible: It is one thing to have everyone around you that needs the best for you; it is something else to allow those individuals to additionally hold you in line! Once in a while, what makes an emotionally supportive network solid and dependable is that they can keep us responsible. They can give us productive criticism that is genuinely to our greatest advantage and will just get us rolling forward better and more grounded. In any case, it begins with you allowing everyone around you to have open and direct discussions with you. It is about you telling them that you invite their viewpoints and criticism for however long it is done non-critically. You don't maintain that your emotionally supportive network should tread lightly for you, reluctant to express what's at the forefront of their thoughts. A sound relationship works in two different ways. So with regards to your emotionally supportive network, it isn't just about the assistance they can give you; it is also about additional input and ideas.

Chapter 5: Self-Awareness and Improvement

You could have gone over the term self-awareness and thought about what it implies. Self-improvement is additionally called personal development and self-development.
What is self-improvement? This term alludes to different strategies for working on one's propensities, conduct, activities, and responses. The following are a couple of guides to explain what self-improvement is:
Figuring out how to control outrage
Figuring out how to beat delaying Figuring out how to conquer apathy Figuring out how to be more amenable and thoughtful
Turning into a more mindful individual Learning new things and growing new abilities Having an impact on your outlook and turning out to be more certain Effective self-awareness requires inspiration, the craving to improve, and the ability to endeavor to make changes. You likewise

should escape your usual range of familiarity and, once in a while, do things that are awkward yet are to your benefit. A receptive outlook and the craving to learn and develop are likewise significant. Self-awareness is a continuous interaction that begins at the beginning and is for the most part molded by guardians, instructors, and the climate. Anyway, to capitalize on it, you really want to become mindful of the interaction, understand what it is, and take the time to develop and work on yourself. In some cases, issues and hardships are the triggers that stir the longing to develop and lead to making changes in one's day-to-day existence. At different times, individuals are propelled to move toward self-improvement subsequent to perusing a motivating book, watching a film, or learning about individuals who have made progress. This frequently drives individuals to new ways, to making changes in their lives, extending their insight and mindfulness, further developing abilities, and growing new ones.

How Would You Learn Self-Improvement?
Self-improvement can help you in all parts
of your life. It can help you at work. It can
change your disposition toward work and,
accordingly, open new doors for headway.
Self-awareness can help in developing
sincerely and intellectually and turning into
a more chivalrous, cherishing, and positive
individual. It can likewise assist you with
seeing your errors and negative propensities
and lead you to rectifying and evolving
them. There are numerous strategies for
self-awareness, like innovative perception,
rehashing certifications, and fostering a
positive outlook and contemplation.
Self-improvement likewise includes guiding,
training, and perusing. An extremely
straightforward and helpful technique for
self-awareness is to check out your way of
behaving and your existence with an open
and fair mind. This will show you what
transformations you really want to make in
yourself and in your life. Seeing how
individuals act can likewise help you. Along

these lines, you can perceive positive and negative attributes of character and become mindful, whether you have or need them, and along these lines, you can realize what you want to work on in yourself. Individuals are unique in relation to each other, and what works for one probably won't work for another. This implies that you should investigate the different procedures and ways for self-improvement to find what is appropriate for you. "Development starts when we start to acknowledge our own shortcomings." Jean Vanier "The main thing that stands between a man and what he needs from life is, much of the time, only the will to attempt it and the confidence to accept that it is conceivable." Richard M. Devotionals

Chapter 6 Balancing Life And Work

Feeling like all you do is work? You're in good company. A few insights show that in excess of 60% of U.S. representatives feel like their balance between fun and serious activities is messed up. Yet, how would you adjust your work-life balance with such a lot of work occurring at home? Also, how would you adjust your responsibility to be more proficient? Is it something beyond hitting a week-after-week yoga class? Furthermore, in particular, in this present reality where the limits between work and home are progressively obscured, how would you sort out what functions? With so many battling to secure concordance between their positions and their home lives, it can appear to be inescapable to feel overpowered and exhausted. Be that as it may, it doesn't need to be. Here we'll distinguish the design of a sound and undesirable balance between serious and fun activities and ways people and supervisors can track down better approaches to overseeing both. What does taking care of business-life balance mean? A sound balance between fun and serious activities alludes to keeping an amicable connection between your work and individual life. It includes intentionally dealing with your significant investment to meet both expert and individual responsibilities while focusing on taking care of oneself and prosperity. In an ideal world, this logic goes: after work, we're ready to invest energy in things that feed us as individuals. This could include investing energy with loved ones or participating in a side interest. A few qualities of a solid balance between serious and fun activities might include: Defining limits: This includes laying out clear limits between work and individual life by characterizing explicit working hours and isolating business-related assignments from individual exercises. Using time effectively: Productively coordinating and focusing on undertakings, guaranteeing that you designate sufficient time for work liabilities as well as special goals, like investing energy with family, participating in leisure activities, or seeking after private objectives Stress the board: Executing techniques to oversee feelings of anxiety, for example, rehearsing care, participating in customary actual work, enjoying reprieves, and turning off from business-related exercises when required Adaptability: Being able to adjust and change your timetable to accommodate unexpected conditions or individual necessities without imperiling work responsibilities Why is the balance between fun and serious activities so significant? Very much like in our weight control plans, to remain solid and stimulated for the long stretch, individuals need assortment. With regards to the balance between serious and fun activities, individuals need to participate in various exercises and rest. We will generally fall into the snare of accepting that we can be useful constantly or that an eight-hour day at work compares to eight hours of result. In any case, that is hard, on the off chance that it is certainly feasible for some people to accomplish. Furthermore, exhaustion has adverse results for the two representatives and bosses. Obsessive workers and individuals who battle to rehearse taking care of themselves end up at a higher risk for burnout, exhaustion, and stress-related medical problems. Unfortunate balance between fun and serious activities can likewise leave representatives working more hours yet being less useful. What is the unfortunate balance between fun and serious activities? Then again, an unfortunate balance between fun and serious activities happens when work becomes overpowering and overshadows individual life, prompting adverse results for a person's prosperity. A few indications of an undesirable balance between serious and fun activities might include: Consistent exhaustion: Consistently working extended periods, including ends of the week and occasions, without adequate time for rest, unwinding, or individual exercises Dismissed individual life: Forfeiting individual connections, side interests, and recreation exercises because of exorbitant work requests Burnout: encountering physical, mental, and close-to-home fatigue because of ongoing pressure and business-related pressure Absence of taking care of oneself: Neglecting to focus on taking care of oneself through exercises like activity, satisfactory rest, and relaxation time bringing about weakening physical and emotional wellness Stressed connections: encountering challenges in keeping up with sound associations with family, companions, and friends and family because of business-related responsibilities Keep in mind that achieving a solid balance between serious and fun activities might change from one individual to another, contingent upon individual conditions and inclinations. It is vital to find an equilibrium that works for you and advances your general prosperity. Indications of an uneven

work-life dynamic An unfortunate balance
between fun and serious activities can have
a far greater effect than simply skirting the
exercise center. One investigation
discovered that the risk of stroke is higher in
individuals who work over 55 hours per
week. A similar measure of work hours is
likewise connected with a higher risk of
uneasiness and gloom. What's more, in any
event, while adapting to genuinely ordinary
rest designs, one more investigation
discovered that functioning longer hours
corresponded with a decrease in actual
wellbeing. By its actual definition, the
balance between fun and serious activities
influences all parts of your life. It will in
general show up contrastingly for various
individuals, be that as it may. The following
are eight qualities related to unfortunate
equilibrium: You can't quit pondering work
when you're not working. Individuals who
find it hard to draw limits between work and
life are at higher risk of burnout. Your
connections—both inside and beyond

work—are starting to endure. You might be handily disturbed with collaborators and far off with friends and family. You feel off. You have unexplained a throbbing pain. You may seldom have energy or find it challenging to concentrate when at work. At the point when you're not working, everything appears to be tiresome or irrelevant. You simply don't want to do anything except if you need to. You frequently turn down solicitations, further segregating yourself from your companions. You burn through a large chunk of change reevaluating support for individual errands. Your clothing, dishes, and mail stack up, sitting tight for the day when you "have the opportunity and willpower" to find time for them. You battle to get some much-needed rest when you're debilitated, intellectually stressed, or when you want to deal with individual errands. You don't recall your last excursion, and you don't have plans to take one. You can't imagine how you will help for the remainder of your life. Regardless of whether you work in a field or an organization you once cherished, it feels difficult to envision proceeding with life, all things considered, for a really long time. You generally feel like, regardless of what you're doing, you ought to accomplish something different. Over the long run, this absence of presence and course frequently prompts an existential emergency. The most effective method to further develop a balance between fun and serious activities Truly, there's no remedy that will fit everybody. Also, you might need to play with what time scale feels generally applicable to you. Attempting to find balance in any single day might feel baffling, yet achieving equilibrium might be simpler to accomplish across possibly more than seven days. The most effective way to decide the best equilibrium for you is by figuring out how to check in with your inward compass—and your outcomes. With deliberateness and a little imagination, you can recalibrate your assumptions and reset

your work-home equilibrium. The following
are 12 hints to have a great balance between
serious and fun activities:
1. Prepare to consolidate work exercises
with relaxation, social, or wellness exercises.
On the off chance that you wind up with a
few virtual gatherings one after the other,
have a go at taking them while you take a
walk. You could likewise accept a call
outside (on the off chance that
encompassing clamor permits!) or, on the
other hand, welcome a companion over to
work with you. 2. Embrace the manner in
which your mind works. Use efficiency
hacks like a Pomodoro clock to work so that
engagement explodes. Shut out any
remaining interruptions so you can take
advantage of your time.
3. Set blocks of time for various
undertakings. Assign an opportunity to
check (and answer) messages, a chance to
take part in gatherings, and a chance to
accomplish intellectually serious work. It
assists with mooring these assignments

around the times that you are becoming more useful.

4. End work at a specific time. There's a platitude that "work extends to occupy the time designated," and when you telecommute, it's much simpler to allow work to pour out into individual time. Put down a point in time to end work for the afternoon, and build up it by shutting down business-related gadgets, locking your office, or planning something a while later.

5. Enroll Innovation to assist you with turning off Utilize an application to impede diverting sites during the day and afterward block work instruments at night. On the off chance that you would be able, limit work to one gadget or attempt to keep one sans work gadget so you can separate totally.

6. Go out for lunch or appreciate lunch with collaborators. Regardless of whether you're telecommuting, you can go out for your mid-day break or associate with partners. The difference in speed will be

reviving—and, obviously, will remind you to eat something as a matter of fact.

7. Get some much-needed rest. At the point when you're home constantly, you will generally attempt to deal with diseases that surely would have kept you home from the workplace. Downtime, including wiped-out time, individual time, excursions, and mourning, are significant ways of sustaining your prosperity.

8. Practice care. Care makes unevenness hard to overlook. At the point when you practice care methods similar to contemplation or breath mindfulness, you become more in line with your feelings and actual sensations. Focusing on these sentiments assists you with figuring out how to see when you may be stifling a need to work. It's difficult to get back to that accounting sheet after you notice your stomach thundering. without a tech break a day.

9. something you love beyond work to take part in Assuming you have something that

you're amped up for accomplishing after work, it will make it more straightforward to detach from work messages or end your day at a foreordained time. Our leisure activities help our energy and essentialness. At the point when we play and feel innovative, we take our new selves back to work.

10. Reexamine work that causes you to long for balance. Assuming your work feels totally irrelevant to the exercises that mix your advantage, excitement, energy, and feeling of importance, you might have to take a gander at how you can change the work you do or the manner in which you make it happen. While work doesn't have to (and can't) fulfill each of your requirements for reason, meaning, social association, and challenge, we can anticipate that work should give snapshots of fulfillment, achievement, and association.

11. Speak with your director. The unfortunate balance between serious and fun activities is, in many cases, exacerbated by the trepidation that we're not doing

what's necessary. Conversing with your chiefs can assist you in focusing on where to invest your energy. Assuming there truly is an excessive amount to do, it very well may be an ideal opportunity to discuss employing extra assistance or smoothing out specific assignments.

12. Work with a mentor or specialist. In the event that you feel overpowered, stuck, or don't have the foggiest idea where to start, working with an expert can be significant. A mentor or instructor can pose the right inquiries and assist you with distinguishing which changes will have the greatest effect and how to get everything rolling. A single word of counsel: begin little. Despite the fact that you might be restless for your balance between serious and fun activities to improve, your work propensities have been worked out over the long run, and logical won't change for the time being. If your objective, for instance, is to decrease screen time, attempting to limit yourself to a specific number of hours will likely

disappoint you. You're bound to stay with another propensity on the off chance that you start with a more modest objective—say, one five-minute 7 different ways administrators can uphold their representatives' balance between serious and fun activities. Doing whatever it takes to foster a sound balance between fun and serious activities can be troublesome. As a supervisor and a compassionate pioneer, you can help your workers (and yourself) by building pathways for them to roll out these improvements. The following are seven different ways supervisors can assist their representatives with building a great balance between serious and fun activities:
1. Remind your group to turn off Urge your group to leave their PCs and work telephones at home when they take some time off. You might figure it doesn't need to be said; however, they will see the value in the unequivocal consent.
2. Give workers space to associate. Sort out virtual blissful hours, birthday celebrations,

book clubs, and different chances to socially interface. Put your mid-day break on your schedule so they can see that you eat as well.
3. Teach representatives their advantages. Remind your workers that wiped-out leave and PTO are important for their pay, and remember to exploit them yourself! With regards to going on vacation, talk is cheap.
4. Check in with direct reports. Make time during your registration to get some information about representative prosperity. You might need to figure out a deeper meaning for what's not being said. Missed cutoff times or an absence of responsiveness can demonstrate overpower.
5. Set a model for your group. Take gatherings while strolling, acquaint them with your children on Zoom (we definitely know they're there), or space out gatherings so they make them inhale room.
6. Know about organizational culture and standards. Make an effort not to standardize a "texting" culture. Clarify that messages sent off-hours don't need quick

consideration, and keep away from deciphering responsiveness as commitment. 7. Regarding working hours: Try not to plan gatherings beforehand or after work hours. This can be interesting while working across various time regions. Urge your representatives to end work at an assigned time every day and check in with anybody you notice reliably working late at night. Finding balance between fun and serious activities while working from a distance One could figure that working remotely would make it more straightforward to achieve a balance between fun and serious activities. Notwithstanding, remote work presents its own difficulties. Working beyond the workplace will in general mean performing multiple tasks, interruptions, and trouble keeping severe hours—all awful news for efficiency as well as keeping work and life discrete. Prior to the COVID pandemic, around 20% of the U.S. labor force telecommuted. Essentially short-term, that number soars to almost 70%. Homes became places for work, school, dinners, recreation, and, surprisingly, working out. There are a few clear potential gains. It's never been more straightforward to carry your own lunch to work; busy time is a relic of days gone by, and it just requires a moment to throw in a heap of clothing before your next gathering. In any case, taking part in numerous exercises in a similar space makes it harder for your cerebrum to recognize work and recreation. We come up short on typical prompts of individuals passing on the workplace to flag when the time has come to wrap up work. When your "office" is at the edge of your room or your lounge area table, it makes it hard to quit contemplating work when work is finished—and simple to browse your email only once again. Furthermore, in spite of the fact that we recover time from a drive, many individuals miss the reality of progressing from home life to endless work life at home. In a period of social removal, our balance between serious and fun activities is currently battling. For some, our work has to a great extent changed in accordance with the pandemic, yet a considerable number of our recreation exercises and most loved outlets have not. Subsequently, it's significantly simpler to get maneuvered into work. We might trust that the gathering with the showcasing group will give a touch of the sought-after friendly cooperation and feeling that we'd typically get at the rec center, a show, or going out with companions. Find and keep a solid balance between fun and serious activities. Finding that the connection between work and home life is wrong is the most vital phase in amending it. It could require some investment, yet little day-to-day or week-after-week propensities can have an enormous effect over the long haul. On the off chance that you really want assistance in working out an arrangement to further develop your balance between serious and fun activities, training can help.

Chapter 7: Monetary Authority

Monetary dominance will require a considerable measure of conceded satisfaction and self-restraint. It is difficult, yet you realize it is completely worth the effort. The excursion can be desolate, except if you encircle yourself with a local area that spurs you and keeps you centered. I paid for the vast majority of my undergrad schooling. I was 17 when I began. I found a new line of work nearby: first in the cleaning group, and afterward as technical support. My cleaning position paid $6.50 or so an hour; however, at that point, I hustled and found the most sought-after work nearby, acquiring $11.11 for 60 minutes. I truly ought to let you know how I hustled that work, yet we should save it for a future section. Until further notice, you want to realize that I made about $3,000 each semester. After charges, the real cash that came into my record was about $2500. Yet, toward the end of each and every semester,

$2100 to $2400 of that cash was utilized to cover my school expenses and educational costs. None of my companions at the time realized that I was paying for school myself. Large numbers of them had caught wind of my astounding nearby work. They had known about the posting, yet hadn't hustled the hustle I hustled to find the work.
The compensation was plainly publicized, so they likewise knew the kind of check I was making. A large number of these companions dealt with grounds as well as gotten payments from their folks. Really, I didn't. As is typical for youngsters at that age, my companions and I needed to appreciate life. They consistently coordinated excursions to the movies, travels to local urban communities, and evenings at the club. In view of my objective to pay my direction through school, I routinely expected to turn down their solicitations to hang making the rounds. At some point, my then-dearest companion went to me and said, "No doubt about it."

This was a person who consistently flaunted about the way that a rich companion of his dad's was paying his educational costs, leaving his father to send him over to the US with heaps of pocket cash. As you can imagine, that kinship didn't keep going for long. It required about a year to completely remove myself from that kinship, yet I unobtrusively exchanged gatherings and became companions with an alternate gathering of folks whose objectives were basically the same as mine. They looked for grants to assist with educational costs; they examined ways of bringing in cash during occasions; they were my clan. As a matter of fact, I was simply on a Zoom call last Saturday with each of them. More than 10 years after the fact, we are still companions. This story shows the dynamic and detached ways your gathering of companions can help you stay on target. A portion of those dynamic ways include: Shared objectives: Your gathering of companions routinely talks about and knows about the way that you are chasing after comparative life objections. Shared exercises: Collectively, you invest your energy getting things done to support that common objective. Persuading discussions: Hearing others discuss their objectives inspires you to genuinely take yours significantly more seriously. Sound contest: Since you see your companions sorting this out, you understand that you would rather not be forgotten about. As Nigerians say, "I can't come and convey last!" However, some of the time, the detached inspiration is significantly more impressive. For example, in my gathering: Positive companion pressure: There was an implicit assumption that we all would be thrifty with our cash. Going a little overboard just wasn't, nevertheless, the gathering's way of life. Irresistible inspiration: At the point when I could have been enticed to forsake my objectives, I was spurred to continue to go on the grounds that I was encircled by other people who were holding themselves to elevated requirements. Self-actualization: Lastly, each time I hit my objective, I had an extraordinary outlook on myself. I was a lot more grounded while managing the following monetary objective. My certainty became unshakeable. Anyway, how would you assemble this local area? On the off chance that you're in your 20s and 30s, almost certainly, you have a central arrangement of companions—individuals that are nearest to you. Investigate the rundown above. Does your ongoing gathering of companions help you in those ways? In the event that the response is no, you really want new companions. Or, on the other hand, you might have to pull closer to the right companions currently in your circle and put a little distance between you and those that are not assisting you with being perfect. Encircle yourself with the perfect individuals; you can and will become together.

Chapter 8: Wellbeing and Health

What Is Wellbeing and Health? Individuals frequently utilize the terms wellbeing and health reciprocally. Although an individual can't have one and not be different, they are two distinct ideas that are very factored, and their implications are unique. The World Wellbeing Association (WHO) characterizes wellbeing as "a condition of complete physical, mental, and social prosperity and not only the shortfall of infection or sickness (disease)." WHO characterizes wellbeing as "the ideal condition of strength for people and gatherings," and health is communicated as "a positive way to deal with living."
The essential contrast between wellbeing and health is that wellbeing is the objective and health is the dynamic course of accomplishing it. You genuinely can't have wellbeing without first achieving health.

Wellbeing impacts, by and large, wellbeing, which is fundamental for living a vigorous, cheerful, and satisfied life. Wellbeing versus health While you can't pick the condition of wellbeing, you can deliberately pick health by carrying on with your life dependably and making proactive strides for your prosperity. Wellbeing involves the determination of a sickness or illness, the inclination toward an illness, and any startling injury. Health is a functioning course of development and change to arrive at your fullest wellbeing and prosperity. It is related to effectively chasing after exercises, simply deciding and making way of life changes, controlling risk factors that can hurt an individual, zeroing in on sustenance, having a reasonable eating routine, and following otherworldly practices that lead to all-encompassing wellbeing. Risk factors are activities or conditions that increase an individual's risk of sickness or injury. A portion of the gambling factors that can be harmful to great wellbeing are as follows:

Smoking is a significant risk factor for cellular breakdown in the lungs and cardiovascular illnesses. Drinking liquor can cause liver harm, strokes, heart infections, and disease. Unprotected sex: It spreads physically transmitted infections, including human immunodeficiency virus (HIV). Outrageous actual work or sports: This might prompt broken bones and different sorts of wounds. What number of aspects of wellbeing are there? Wellbeing is something beyond actual wellbeing; it is all-encompassing and multi-faceted. It involves six aspects that incorporate physical, scholarly, close-to-home, ecological, social, and profound wellbeing. Physical: Actual wellbeing increments actual wellness—by being in great shape, an individual would have an improved capacity to forestall sickness and illnesses. Practice invigorates a sound psyche and body. A stationary way of life can be tried not to by increasing active work in day-to-day existence like strolling, cycling, strolling the canine, making strides, and climbing. Having great nourishment, eating a decent eating regimen, drinking adequate water (eight glasses each day), and getting sufficient rest advance an individual's actual wellbeing. Intellectual: Mental activity and commitment through learning, critical thinking, and innovativeness support scholarly wellbeing and advance a superior disposition. Individuals who learn new things and challenge their psyche can stay away from psychological well-being issues. Emotional: An individual with close-to-home health can manage upsetting circumstances. An individual who knows about their own sentiments, has great confidence, and has compassion toward others' sentiments would have profound wellbeing. Environmental: Familiarity with the job we play in further developing our common habitat as opposed to criticizing it and keeping up with and living in a solid actual climate liberated from dangers advances health. Social: Groups of friends and encouraging groups of people are priceless to the general prosperity of an individual. Relating, connecting, and adding to a local area, laying out great relational relations, and keeping up with long-term associations with loved ones make an individual more joyful and better. Spiritual: Otherworldly wellbeing doesn't infer religion or confidence in an individual, yet the quest for significance and motivation behind human life Creating sympathy, being mindful, pardoning, and having a reason in life help with profound wellbeing. This can be accomplished through contemplation, charitable effort, investing energy in nature, and so on. On the one hand, patients with chronic weakness draw on the clinical organization to treat diseases. On the opposite end, individuals center proactively around avoidance and boost their imperativeness. They take on ways of life that further develop wellbeing, forestall infection, and upgrade their personal satisfaction and a feeling of prosperity.

Wellbeing is proactive, preventive, and driven by self-obligation regarding solid living. Does your body run best on 8 glasses of water a day? Not really. Everybody has different liquid necessities. The climate—both temperature and stickiness—has an impact, as do your size, orientation, and level of action. Things being what they are, are 8 glasses of water a day truly connected with great wellbeing? Some say 8 glasses of water assist with weight reduction. That wasn't valid for 38 overweight and corpulent adolescents, however, who were approached by analysts to hydrate for a very long time. Those analysts tracked down no connection between drinking 8 glasses of water and weight reduction. Others guarantee that drinking additional water beyond what you're eager for helps hydrate or smooth skin, lessens cerebral pains, or helps flush additional poisons from the kidneys. These cases were painstakingly explored and viewed as false: "There is no obvious proof of advantage from drinking expanded measures of water," the analysts concluded. All things being equal, this investigation discovered that drinking when parched is adequate for the vast majority. Are eggs connected to high blood cholesterol? Eggs pack bunches of cholesterol, compared with different food sources. Cholesterol in the blood is emphatically connected with coronary illness and cardiovascular failures. All in all, eating heaps of eggs ought to be awful for your heart, isn't that so? It appears to be valid, yet most dietary examinations say something else. Upwards of one egg each day doesn't raise your risk of cardiovascular sickness, which can prompt respiratory failure, for individuals with ordinary cholesterol. That could be on the grounds that eggs have other heart-safeguarding properties beyond cholesterol. It might likewise be on the grounds that eating cholesterol is just feebly connected with bringing cholesterol up in your blood. Whatever the explanation, your egg propensity most likely won't hurt your heart whenever done with some restraint. Is antiperspirant connected to bosom malignant growth or Alzheimer's infection? Those fears went out to both be unwarranted. Over quite a while back, alerts were being rung in the wellbeing scene connected with antiperspirants and dementia. Scientists tracked down higher proportions of aluminum in the minds of Alzheimer's patients. There were fears that the aluminum that briefly plugs your perspiration channels could raise the dangers of neurological issues. In any case, over the long run, no proof has arisen to help this. All things considered, it appears that Alzheimer's psychologists are in your mind, abandoning a higher centralization of aluminum. What's more, it appears that the aluminum in an antiperspirant is scarcely consumed by your skin. At the end of the day, aluminum in the cerebrum is by all accounts an outcome of Alzheimer's and not a reason, and antiperspirants presumably raise no risk of dementia, including Alzheimer's. It was inadequately grasped science that began the Alzheimer's panic; however, a junk email was liable for persuading parts regarding ladies during the 1990s that their antiperspirant was raising their gamble of bosom malignant growth. The email erroneously asserts that antiperspirants trap unsafe synthetic substances inside your body. It turns out the entirety of your underarm antiperspirant blocks are sweat and body salt. What eliminates the more harmful poisons in your body? Your pee and excrement do. What's more, there is no reality to this clinical fantasy; the American Malignant Growth Society says there is no connection between antiperspirants and bosom disease. Cold air causes colds. You might have heard this one from your mom: "Try not to go outside with wet hair or you'll contract a bug!" With all due regard to Mother, that isn't the manner in which colds are spread. Assuming you go outside in a chilly climate, regardless of wet

garments or hair, you stand no more serious
risk of coming down with a bug. Colds come
from infections, and infections can be
spread no matter what the climate. For what
reason do colds and sicknesses turn out to
be so normal in the colder time of year? The
facts confirm that there is a "cool season"
and an "influenza season" that endures from
about October to May. However, why? One
hypothesis is that a chilly climate powers
individuals inside, where cold and seasonal
infections spread all the more effectively in a
closed space where individuals are clustered
together.

Might you at any point detoxify your body?
Does your body require a purge to flush
itself of poisons? The idea is engaging. In
the event that you could free your
assemblage of terrible synthetics that could
give you more energy, mental concentration,
or better rest, couldn't you make it happen?
Additionally, there's something fulfilling
about removing awful things from your
body, particularly in the event that you're

told it will fix another medical condition. So does detoxifying your body work? For specialists to be aware that a detoxification treatment works, they need to know two things. In the first place, they need to understand what poison is being eliminated from the body. Second, they need to know how it will be eliminated. A gathering of researchers explored 15 items that could detoxify your body. The items went from face wipes to filtered water. A large portion of the organizations selling these items essentially renamed standard cycles like cleaning or brushing, referring to them as "detoxifying." For instance, one of those faces cleans "detoxified" soil and cosmetics—precisely what you would anticipate that any facial scour should do. The specialists said these organizations could neither make sense of how they eliminated poisons nor what "poisons" their items were intended to eliminate. All in all, they basically utilized "detox" as a trendy expression. So in the event that an item professes to scrub your colon, chelate your kidneys, or assist you with working out poisons, reconsider buying. Real detoxification occurs in an emergency clinic, and generally just when something has truly turned out badly, as in patients with weighty metal harming or the clinical treatment of a drunkard. Might extraordinary items at any point lift your resistant framework? Numerous items guarantee to improve or "support" your resistant framework here and there. However, they will more often than not be fluffy on the points of interest. You ought to ask yourself, "Which piece of the resistant framework does it support?" Your safe framework is a complicated series of cycles, including antibodies, certain proteins, portions of your blood (counting white platelets), and considerably more. At the point when an item just says it "supports resistance" yet doesn't say how, that ought to raise a warning. Additionally, there are ways your resistance framework can be raised that would be destructive to your body. One of the main parts of your safe capability is irritation, the regular cycle your body sanctions to fend off microorganisms, infections, and anything in your body that your cells don't perceive as a piece of your body. Initiating your incendiary reaction is one way an item can support your safe framework, yet it would likewise be helping your risk of stroke, coronary failure, and other medical conditions. Your absolute best shot at further developing your safe reaction is to follow the wellbeing nuts and bolts: get a lot of rest, work out consistently, and eat quality food sources. Indeed, even there, research is progressing and a lot of debate remains. You Just Utilize 10% of Your Cerebrum? Assuming you just utilized 10% of the cerebrum, does that mean you could eliminate 90% and be fine? Individuals who support this normal case say that assuming you had the option to utilize the remainder of your psychological power, you could open gigantic capacities concealing profound inside. The main difficulty? It's not, by any stretch of the imagination, valid. It may be the case that 1930s rodents prompted this thought. In these examinations, portions of rodents' cerebrums were eliminated, and the rodents may as yet perform fundamental undertakings. Yet, that was just a particular piece of the rodents' cerebrums, and the rodents might have had different inadequacies that weren't tried. Any place the fantasy came from, it stays a legend. Cerebrum checks obviously show that regardless of what movement you make, your mind is dynamic and locked in. Of course, a few pieces of the cerebrum are "turned on" for certain exercises more than others; however, there aren't any regions that aren't utilized. Does swimming just subsequent to eating give you spasms? How long would it be advisable for you to hold on to swim in the wake of eating? The exhortation to stand by in the wake of eating has been around for no less than 100 years, for the most part with the advance notice that you will seize up assuming you swim too early. Luckily for youthful swimmers all over, there is no reality to this normal wellbeing fantasy. Be that as it may, imagine a scenario in which you really do get a spasm while swimming. Regardless of whether a full stomach won't cause it, you could pull a muscle while you swim or get a cramp. Squeezing won't make you sneak by the water, as long as you don't overreact. In the event that you, in all actuality, do begin to squeeze while you swim, fix and loosen up the confined muscle until the issue figures out its direction.

Chapter 9 Celebrating success

Praise for an achievement like a commemoration, a birthday, or an extraordinary arrangement of grades can give us an astonishing inclination. Furthermore, it very well may be far and away superior when another person sees our accomplishments and makes an attempt to recognize them. This is valid and working as well. Commending accomplishments can support certainty and increase inspiration. Showing appreciation can likewise support your association's standing, further develop maintenance, and assist with drawing in top talent.

Be that as it may, how much acknowledgment is sufficient? Furthermore, when do festivities become oppressive or lose meaning? In this article, we investigate nine methods for praising accomplishment in your group while keeping away from the entanglements.

Observing Achievement Pause for a minute to consider how your group or association praises achievement or accomplishment. Is it having a positive effect? In a study by the American Mental Affiliation (APA), most respondents said that their organizations worked on some sort of acknowledgment plot. In any case, in excess of 33% of individuals overviewed had gotten no acknowledgment in the earlier year. Not exactly half said that acknowledgment was given decently, and just half said that they felt esteemed by their boss. The business presumably had good motivations, yet these plans were possible a misuse of exertion and assets and left numerous representatives feeling disheartened instead of propelled. On the off chance that you celebrate accomplishment in the correct manner, you'll probably build certainty and inspiration, prompting more joyful and useful groups. Assuming you seldom recognize a wonderful piece of handiwork (or you celebrate one that feels constrained, uncalled for, or improper), there's a gamble that resolve and devotion will get away. A standing for praising successes and exertion can likewise turn into a focal mainstay of your manager's marking, assisting your association with drawing in and holding ability. What Is Accomplishment? At the point when we consider an accomplishment, we will generally picture something strange, such as surpassing targets, handling a major deal, or conveying an undertaking achievement. Yet, other, less quantifiable, ways of behaving merit acknowledgment as well—for instance, arranging collectively to head off an emergency, mastering and applying another expertise, or supporting newcomers. Indeed, even something really basic is deserving of festivity. You could ask why you ought to try to support your colleagues' confidence in any case. All things considered, would they confirm or deny that they are simply doing what they're paid for? However, confident groups don't "become complacent." Recognizing and commending their accomplishments is important for building a compelling, driven group that will effectively look to further develop results and execution. Make Festivity Significant Whatever you decide to celebrate, ensure it's fitting for the individuals included. A festival can take many forms, from a private, relaxed discussion to a public occasion, with no cost saved. Yet, the APA review we alluded to before likewise showed that a prize or gift makes no certain difference on the off chance that the beneficiary doesn't really need it, regardless of the amount you've spent on it. In this way, make certain to consider cautiously your partners' inclinations and characters—and the elements of the group—before you hold a festival. For instance, on the off chance that the individual concerned is a self-observer, they might not have any desire to stand up and give a discourse or get a gift before their partners. All things being equal, a peaceful, individual "great" could be all they need, and they'll see the value in it significantly, seriously realizing that you've considered their inclinations. Likewise, don't present a container of champagne to an individual who doesn't drink liquor or sort out a costly trip for the group when compensations are frozen. Certain individuals might feel irritated or belittled by any plain enthusiasm for their work. According to their point of view, it could appear to infer shock that they've gotten along nicely! There could likewise be a more extensive social blunder to stay away from in the event that you're essential for a socially different group. Likewise, think about whether your association or individuals in your group place more value on outward or natural prizes. For instance, a scrupulous colleague could partake in the valuable chance to invest energy in an individual task rather than getting a financial reward. One method for figuring out what your family values is to just ask them. You can do this casually or through a representative fulfillment review. Remember to praise your own achievements as well! Carve out the opportunity to contemplate what you've accomplished as a component of your own objective setting. This can support your confidence and your feeling of independence and dominance. It can likewise expand your perceivability, especially assuming that you share the credit with others. In any case, try not to enjoy uproarious self-advancement; it might seem like self-importance, your colleagues will not see the value in it, and it could harm your standing. Nine Methods for Observing Accomplishment All in all, how might you recognize and commend achievement? The following are nine choices, which can all be customized to your group's particular necessities. 1. Simply say it. A clear, eye-to-eye "great" is a basic but successful method for commending accomplishment. An individual email can be adequate as well, and a handwritten card or note can add a significant individual touch. Assembling the group to recognize achievement can be a strong proclamation, and a show of approval can be inspiring and group-building; however, take care not to humiliate anybody. 2. Share examples of overcoming adversity. A gathering message is another choice. Tailor it to the particular individual and their accomplishments, yet don't abuse this strategy, or it could seem to be predictable. You can utilize email, the organization pamphlet, web-based entertainment, or an informing stage to share and celebrate examples of overcoming adversity. You might really set up a dedicated channel to feature and praise individuals for unparalleled pieces of handiwork. This has the additional advantage of raising your colleague's profile. 3. Show proactive kindness. While you're praising your very own accomplishment, show your appreciation by recognizing individuals who assisted with getting it going. Continuously pay special attention to valuable chances to assist others with succeeding, so they have motivation to celebrate as well. What's more, when colleagues share uplifting news, they consistently attempt to emphatically answer. Encouraging comments further enhance camaraderie. 4. Give a gift. A celebratory gift could be an oddball cash reward or a non-cash one, like a retail or experience voucher. Cash is often the most well-known reward, yet ponder how different representatives could see it. Remember that some colleagues may, as of now, be boosted with cash rewards. Attempt to try not to start a trend; you don't maintain that acknowledgment should turn out to be only a generic money exchange. Gifts, for example, food or blossoms, are a moderately reasonable yet strong approach to perceiving accomplishment. Ensure that you consider any dietary or sensitivity issues. There may likewise be socially responsive qualities around giving gifts that you ought to know about. 5. Get together socially. Praising by purchasing colleagues a feast or drink can be a viable method for remunerating them and helping camaraderie. In any case, be careful with barring any individual who, for instance, is away on an extended get-away, has extraordinary dietary prerequisites, or has providing care liabilities. On the off chance that you hold your occasion during the functioning day, be aware of partners' cutoff times and be clear about whether you anticipate that they should get back to work a while later. 6. Coordinate a group day out. An excursion to the movies, a feast at an eatery, going to a game, or even a day of open-air exercises are well-known approaches to celebrating. Be that as it may, there are possible dangers to remember as well. Everybody will probably have an alternate thought of "fun," so attempt to find an action that will be famous no matter how you look at it. You won't maintain that anybody should be despondent or decline to partake. This is a specific gamble with physical or open-air exercises that may be challenging for certain individuals for wellbeing, openness, or certainty reasons.

Whenever you've settled on a reasonable occasion, further inquiries to respond to may be: What's remembered for the day to the organization's detriment? Is there anybody who'd find it hard to manage the cost of different pieces of the day? Could individuals bring relatives? Provided that this is true, will those relatives need to take care of themselves? Where does that leave partners who are single or without kids? 7. Offer additional occasions. Time off can be an incredible prize, particularly when your group has worked additional hours to finish an undertaking. Be that as it may, could burning the midnight oil every so often without a great explanation likewise be considered an accomplishment? Be cautious about making bogus assumptions about what's to come. 8. Set up a corridor of popularity. An "representative of the week" noticeboard or warning can be well known and viable; however, it can lose influence over the long haul. You risk allegations of posturing by assuming that you feel obliged to pick somebody instead of nobody, regardless of whether they merit it. What's more, in the event that you continue to perceive a "star" colleague or continually ignore another, you could begin to estrange individuals. 9. Have an honors service. A spectacular night of music, prizes, and talks is a thrilling method for joining mingling, group construction, and coordinating with formal acknowledgment and festivity. On the off chance that you have the spending plan, you can enlist a setting and an expert occasions group. Nonetheless, to restrict the cost and increase cooperation, get your group associated with overseeing and running the occasion, including making the food and outfits. This will be fun and compensating in itself! This rundown is in no way, shape, or form comprehensive. Utilize your creative mind and judgment to make your own festivals, and see what befalls efficiency and occupation fulfillment when your kin feel celebrated and perceived for their work.

Chapter10 Give Back and Impact

Imagine a world where every individual, driven by a sense of compassion and purpose, actively contributes to the well-being of others and the greater good. This world is within our reach, and it's the world envisioned in Chapter 11. Giving back is a transformative power that not only changes the lives of those you help but also enriches your own.
When you give back, you participate in a profound act of kindness and generosity. Whether through financial contributions, volunteer work, advocacy, or social entrepreneurship, you become a beacon of hope, creating positive ripples in the lives of individuals, communities, and even entire societies.
Forms of Giving Back
1. Philanthropy: Philanthropy involves contributing financially to causes and organizations that align with your values and vision. Your financial support can fuel

impactful initiatives, from funding educational programs to supporting medical research or addressing environmental concerns.

2. Volunteering: Volunteering is a hands-on way to make a difference. It's the act of giving your time, skills, and energy to support charitable organizations, community projects, or humanitarian efforts. Volunteering allows you to directly engage with the people and communities you're passionate about helping.

3. Social Entrepreneurship: Social entrepreneurs are change-makers who create businesses with a mission to address social or environmental issues. They blend entrepreneurship with a commitment to creating positive change, tackling problems with innovative solutions.

4. Advocacy and Activism: Advocacy involves using your voice and influence to promote change. Whether you're advocating for human rights, environmental conservation, or social justice, your efforts

can drive awareness and encourage policy changes

Finding Your Passion in Giving Back

To make your impact meaningful and sustainable, it's essential to align your philanthropic efforts with your passions and values. Ask yourself what issues tug at your heartstrings, what causes resonate deeply with you, and where you believe your contributions can have the most significant impact.

Are you passionate about education and its potential to transform lives? Perhaps you're deeply concerned about environmental sustainability or committed to supporting underprivileged communities. Your unique passions and values will guide you toward the causes where your efforts will make the most profound difference.

The Ripple Effect of Impact

Every act of kindness and generosity has the potential to create a ripple effect, extending far beyond its initial impact. When you give back, you inspire others to join your cause or initiate their own efforts for positive change. Your actions serve as a catalyst for a chain reaction of goodwill and progress.

Creating a Legacy

Your commitment to giving back can extend beyond your lifetime. In this chapter, we explore strategies for creating a philanthropic legacy. Whether through endowed foundations, charitable trusts, or other forms of planned giving, you can ensure that your impact continues for generations to come. This legacy becomes a testament to your values and vision, leaving an enduring mark on the world.

Personal Fulfillment through Giving

The act of giving back not only benefits others and society but also brings personal fulfillment and a profound sense of purpose. It allows you to connect with your deepest values, cultivate empathy, and experience the joy that comes from making a meaningful difference in the lives of others. Giving back is a powerful source of

happiness and contentment, contributing to
your overall well-being